# PUTTING ON THE ARMOR OF GOD:

A Survival Handbook for
The Great Awakening
and New Earth.

Copyright © 2021 by Isabella Young
First published
All rights reserved. No part of this book may be reproduced or used in any manner without written permission of the copyright owner except as permitted by U.S. copyright l;aw. Images from Pixabay and the author. For permissions, contact; isabellayoung19@gmail.com
This publication contains the ideas and opinions of its author. It is sold with the understanding that the author and publisher is sharing personal opinions intended to support the reader. to take full responsibility for him/herself.
Published by Isabella Young
ISBN 979-8-9852771-0-4

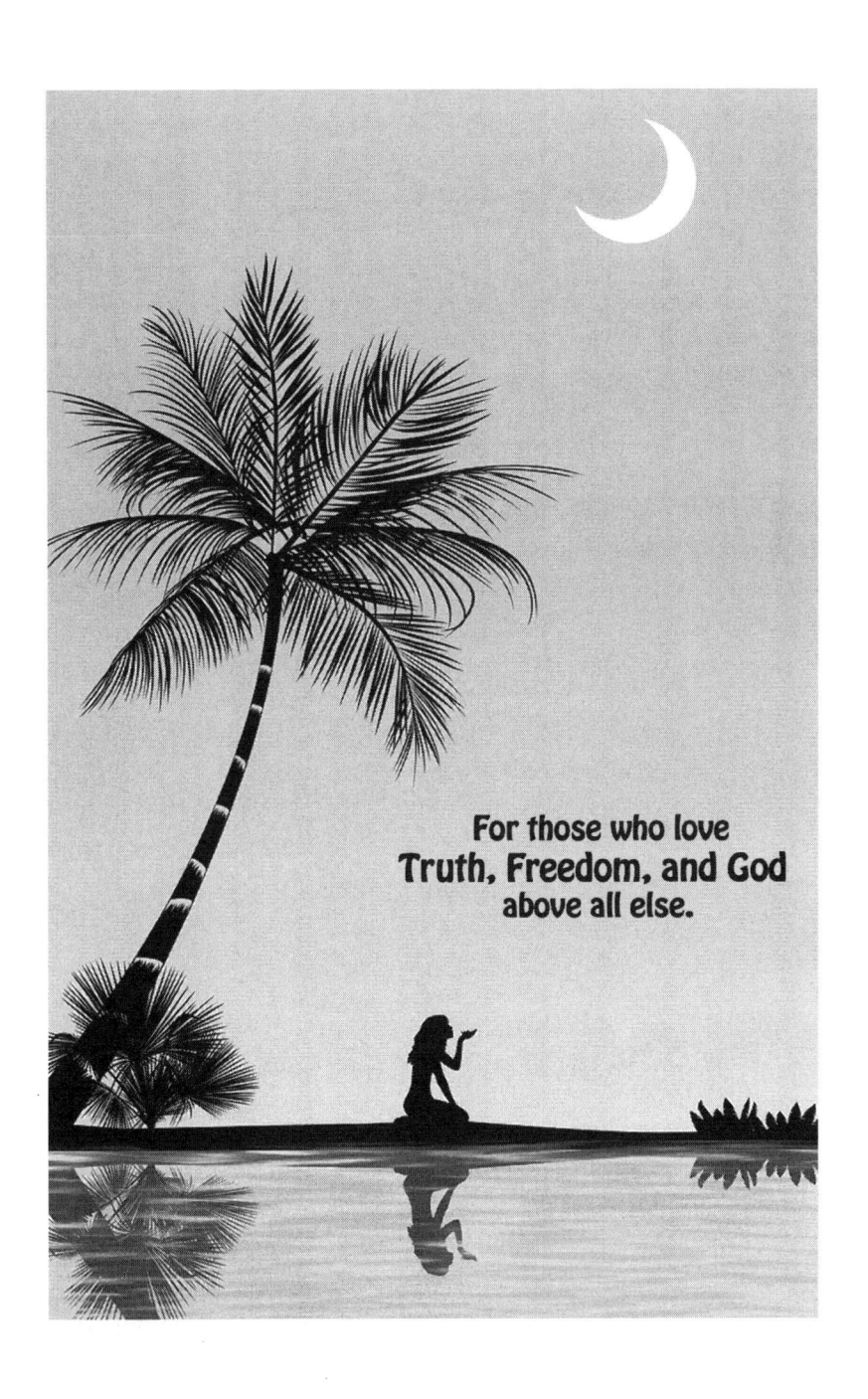

For those who love
**Truth, Freedom, and God**
above all else.

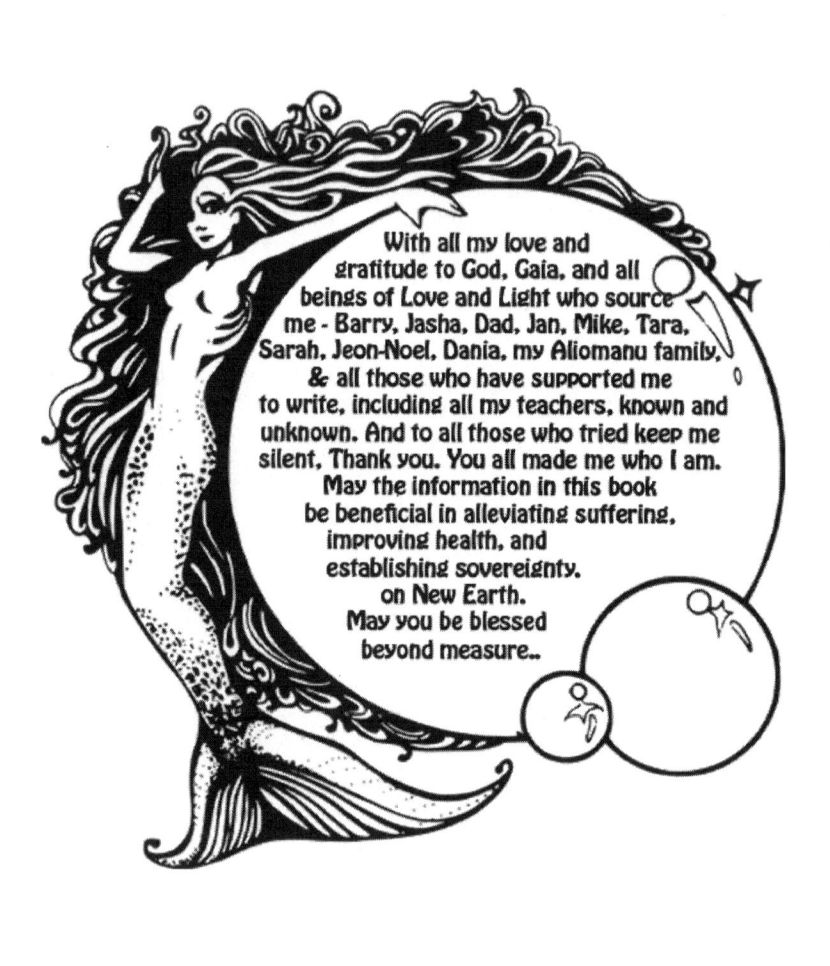

With all my love and gratitude to God, Gaia, and all beings of Love and Light who source me - Barry, Jasha, Dad, Jan, Mike, Tara, Sarah, Jeon-Noel, Dania, my Aliomanu family, & all those who have supported me to write, including all my teachers, known and unknown. And to all those who tried keep me silent, Thank you. You all made me who I am. May the information in this book be beneficial in alleviating suffering, improving health, and establishing sovereignty. on New Earth. May you be blessed beyond measure..

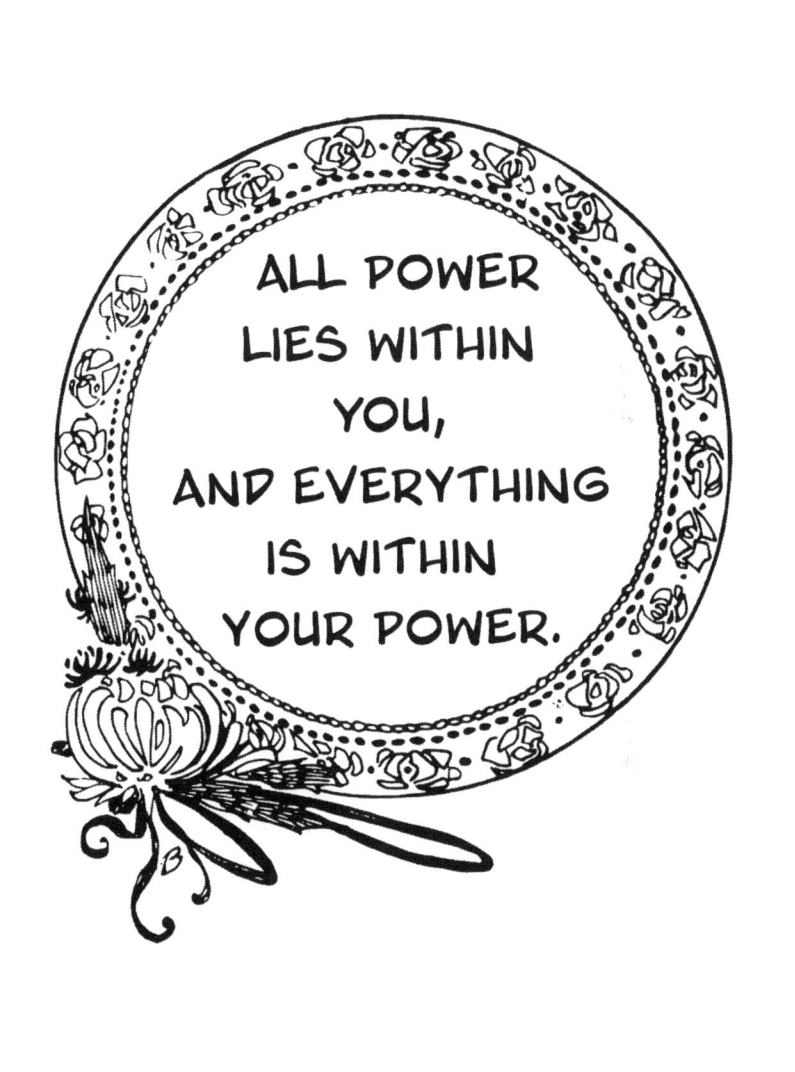

ALL POWER
LIES WITHIN
YOU,
AND EVERYTHING
IS WITHIN
YOUR POWER.

# CONTENTS

| | |
|---|---|
| **INCREASING PERSONAL POWER** | **5** |
| Increasing Spiritual Power | 37 |
| Natural Law | 40 |
| What to Avoid | 66 |
| Increasing Mental Power | 77 |
| Actions to strengthen Will Power | 82 |
| What to Avoid | 91 |
| Increasing Physical Power | 99 |
| What to Avoid | 128 |
| Optimizing Financial Power | 143 |
| What to Avoid | 145 |
| Increasing Personal Power | 146 |
| What to Avoid | 148 |
| Optimizing Personal Power | 148 |
| Co-creating New Earth | 149 |
| | |
| **A VISION FOR NEW EARTH: TERRA NOVA** | **163** |
| Signs and Evidence of New Earth | 175 |
| The Great Rebellion is well underway | 180 |
| The Great Resignation has begun | 181 |
| Resources | 189 |

*There has never been a more important time
to put on the armor of God.
There has never been a more crucial time
to fortify and increase personal power and practice
peaceful dissent.
Attacks upon our health, our sovereignty,
our humanity, our Divinity, and our children
have escalated, and the freedom and future of
humankind are at stake.
We stand between danger and opportunity; lies
and Truth; confusion and clarity; fear and freedom;
powerlessness and infinite power; the old world of
slavery and suffering and the new world of Love,
peace, and freedom.
It is the time of bifurcation, and one must choose:
Love. Unity. Peace. Freedom. Healing.
Consciousness.*

**OR**

*Fear. Division. Anger. Hatred. Greed. Control. A.I.
Everybody will get what they choose.
For those who choose love, there is no time to lose
if we are to come together as an
invincible army of Love/Light
to participate in our evolutionary reality,
and the co-creation of New Earth.*

Knowledge is power, wisdom is freedom, and ignorance is powerlessness. It is not possible to be powerful without awareness of hidden adversaries. It is not possible to be empowered without knowing all the ways personal power is being depleted. It is not possible to be free without knowing that one is being held captive. One of the gifts of the COVID-19 event is the ongoing exposure of evidence and personal experiences that prove that we are being severely disempowered, we are not free, and we are not safe. We are under attack. And a leap of understanding is required to know that it is not from a virus.

> *"For we wrestle not against flesh and blood, but against principalities, against powers of the air, against the rulers of the darkness of this world, against spiritual hosts of wickedness in high places."*
> – EPHESIANS 6:12

Humanity is under attack through physical warfare, psychological warfare, and spiritual warfare. Our enemy has been hidden in plain sight for eons – in the shadows, in unholy alliances, and invisible – controlling human beings through secret societies, black magic, and social engineering using mind control technologies,[1] behavior modification programs,[2]

---

[1] Mind control technologies include television, radios, computers, the Internet, cell phones, movies, music, frequencies, subliminal acoustic manipulation, voice-to-skull technologies, language, symbols, logos, drugs, and implants.

[2] Behavior modification and brainwashing programs include religions,

and psychological warfare strategies to weaken, confuse, and divide us. Weaponry includes fear, trauma-based mind control, social conditioning, propaganda, psyops,[3] black ops, interferometry, confuscation and obfuscation of information, gaslighting, subliminal programming, predictive programming, ideological subversion, controlled opposition, and the Hegelian Dialectic – the Divide and Rule strategy.[4] A tragic public event or crisis is orchestrated, which generates the required public reaction for implementation of a pre-selected solution that progressively erodes human rights, civil liberties, and freedom. Every staged and false-flag event moves us closer to totalitarianism – a One World government and the total enslavement of Humanity.

***Truth is rising like a bubble
through the sea of confusion.***

---

government, politics, banking, corporations, public education, scientism, military and police forces, man's laws, the "Entertainment/Entrainment" industry, Hollywood, pornography, advertising, fashion, the beauty myth, mass media, social media, video games, virtual realities, sports, gambling, popular music, music videos, literature, and carnism (meat eating).

[3] Psychological Operations (Psyops): Psychological operations are operations (staged events) that convey selected information and indicators to people to influence their emotions, motives, objective reasoning, and worldview, and ultimately the behavior of governments, organizations, groups, and individuals. Source: Wikipedia. Recent examples include World Wars, the Moon Landing, 9/11, Global Warming/Climate Change, Earth shape, presidential assassinations, mass shootings, Q, BLM, Antifa, and COVID-19.

[4] Divisions amongst us are reinforced by gender, race, nationality, religions, politics, worldview schisms, medical status, and pronouns.

A fierce battle is being waged beneath the surface of Nature and within every human being beyond cognition and above sensory perception, and it is on this battlefield that we need to achieve our freedom. To be unaware of this war will bring Humanity into its greatest decline. Know thy enemy. The true identity of our enemy has yet to be revealed, but they are "The Hierarchy Enslaving You."[5] They are nonhuman, subhuman, and antihuman. They are soulless, shapeshifting parasites of pure evil, infused and suffused through aristocracy, governments, police and military forces, banks, corporations, mass media, entertainment, sports, and all religious, academic, scientific, and philanthropic institutions. They are the greatest threat to humankind today.

> *"We now live in a world where doctors destroy health, lawyers destroy justice, universities destroy knowledge, governments destroy freedom, the press destroys information, religion destroys morals, and banks destroy the economy."*
> - CHRIS HEDGES

---

[5] They are also known as the Antichrist. Lucifer. Hasatan. Satan. The Devil. The Beast. The Dark Lord. The Serpent. Ba'al. Baphomet. Molech. Mammon. Ahriman. Evil aliens. The Reptilians. Team Lizard. Nephilim. Dracos. Snakeheads. The Devastators. The Tormentors. The Regressives. The Illuminati. The Global Elite. The Cabal. Freemasons. Imposters of Light. Mother of All Vampires. Spirits of Darkness. Dark Reality. Dark Occult. Babylonian Priesthood. Satanic Pharaonic Bloodline. The Black Brotherhood. The Black Hats. The Deep State. Globalists. The Establishment. The 1%. The Shadow Government. The 13 Bloodlines. Committee of 300. The Fourth Reich. The Nazi Hydra. The Ultrazionist cult.The Satanic Blood Cult. The Death Cult. The Beast System. One World Government. New World Order. The Powers That Should Not Be. The Powers That Were.

They are waging the Third World War upon us. It is a non-linear war, and the aim is not to win. The aim is to continue to grow Evil, harness human consciousness, possess souls, prevent the Great Awakening, and control the evolutionary timeline of Humanity using fear-based mind control, perception management, orchestrated conflicts, and confuscation of information to create a constant vaudeville of contradictory narratives that induce fear and confusion, which disempower, divide, intimidate, and control the population. Reality is being presented as bewildering theatre, so no-one is ever sure about what is happening, or what is real and what is fake, and what is true and what is not. In this strange and unsettling time, when nothing makes coherent sense, it is exceedingly difficult for any real opposition with a coherent narrative and a united front to emerge.

*United we stand. Divided we fall.*
*Together we are indivisible and invincible.*
*Nothing is impossible when we are united.*

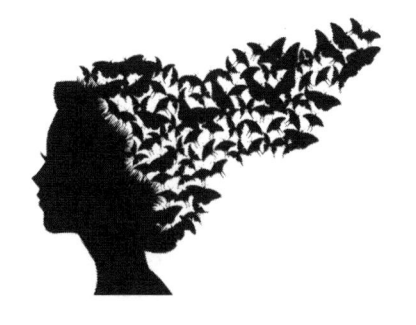

Understanding that Humanity is under attack from a predator species that seeks to suck the lifeblood out of us is central to increasing personal power. Without the knowledge that humankind has an enemy that is holding most human beings captive as loosh[6] in an invisible mind control matrix, we remain powerless. Only with the awareness that we are living in captivity, in a cage for consciousness, can we choose to refuse to be willing captives and free ourselves. The United States of America is not currently the Land of the Free or the Brave, but it will be when we take courageous action to become fully empowered and free ourselves from the tyranny of Evil. Behold the contagion of courage spreading across the world.

> ***"None are more hopelessly enslaved than those who falsely believe they are free."***
> – Johann Wolfgang von Goethe

For those choosing to dismiss the enslavement of Humanity through the manipulation of human consciousness as a "conspiracy theory," please consider the fact that there is always a lot more going on besides the passing pageantry that is being reported or that can be perceived. There are invisible forces above and below our field of awareness that are acting upon us. There are interpenetrating dimensions and unseen forces far greater than those that can be seen.[7] There are countless unseen, intelligent, benevolent, and malevolent beings; celestial bodies; endless realms, dimensions, and

---

[6] First described by Robert Moore, 'loosh' is the energy of human and animal suffering that feeds parasitic lifeforms.

[7] Dimensions are levels of consciousness that vibrate at a certain rate. Each dimension vibrates at a higher rate than the one below it. In each higher dimension, there exists a clearer, expanded perspective of reality and a greater depth of knowing. Most humans perceive less than 1% of reality.

hierarchies; infinite timelines and probabilities; other battles and agendas; and unknown layers of Life to perceive, comprehend, and discover.

***The biggest and most successful conspiracy has been convincing the public that there is no conspiracy.***

What else explains the continuous devolution of our species?

Instead of evolving into a more humane, refined species flourishing on Earth, the crown jewel of the Cosmos, humankind is regressing into a more inhumane, narcissistic, neurotic, psychopathic, self-destructive species. There are perpetual wars, and suffering is endless. Instead of living peacefully, in harmony with the Earth, enjoying the abundance of Earth (which includes food, housing, and free energy for all), and creating beauty and harmony, we are witnessing escalating violence and divisiveness – a cancerous military industrial complex, anti-human artificial/alien intelligence (AI), nuclear weaponry, rigged financial markets, and a secret space program driving economic and geopolitical instability.

We are witnessing obscene greed and materialism drive unsustainable economic growth widening wealth disparity, overconsumption of finite resources, and the horrors of powering the planet on fuels that are killing us and our ecosystem. There is overlogging, overmining, and overfishing. Monoculture and deadly chemical (agrochemical) agriculture. We breath toxic air and ingest toxic foods, drinks, and drugs. We are subject to incessant noise pollution, frequency manipulation, and 5G networks. We are witnessing incomprehensible biodiversity loss. The insect holocaust. Ecocide.

There are local genocides and global genocide. Famines. Poverty. Starvation. Refugees. Mass murderers. Rapists. Pedophiles. Pedevores. Terrorists. Racists. Misogynists. Sadists. Satanists. We live with gender inequality, systematic emasculation and demonization of men, and degradation and exploitation of women and children. Over-medicalization and brutalization of childbirth. Normalization of cesareans, bottle feeding, and early separation of children from family. Employment orphans. The intentional breakdown of the family unit is causing multigenerational traumas and debilitating mental and physical illnesses. There is cultural subversion, ideological infiltration, moral relativism,[8] and moral decline. Systemic political, religious, financial, legal, scientific, medical, academic, philanthropic, and corporate corruption. Capitalism. Consumerism. Censorship. The illusion of choice. The dumbing down of the population. Agnotology. Devolution and debasement of Arts, Science, Literature, Language, and Music. The collapse of reason. The decline of supersensible cognition. The pandemic of cognitive dissonance. The dementia tsunami. Institutionalization, overmedication, and scrapheaping of elders. The pandemic of narcissism. Menticide.

---

[8] Moral Relativism is the ideology that Objective Morality does not exist in Nature, and that "Right" and "Wrong" are merely subjective constructs, which human beings may invent and arbitrate according to time, location, circumstance, or preference.

There is criminalization of entheogens[9] and other natural medicines and cures. Suppressed healing technologies. Weaponized medicine. Medical tyranny. Medical apartheid. Illegal green passes and vaccine passports. Record deaths from foods, pharmaceutical drugs, and iatrogenic illnesses (medical malpractice).[10] Addictions to prescription and non-prescription drugs destroying lives, families, and communities. Malnutrition. The obesity epidemic. Lifespan exceeding healthspan. The autism epidemic. Vaccine holocausts. Forced experimentation. The fertility crisis.[11] Escalating perversions and distortions of sexual energy. Sexualization of children. Systemic child sexual abuse. Millions of missing children. Human trafficking. Human slavery. Adrenochrome farms.[12]

---

[9] An entheogen is a psychoactive substance that is used in a sacred context to induce an altered state of consciousness. It acts as a consciousness-expanding, boundary-dissolving agent that facilitates the experience of unity consciousness, Oneness, Divine Love, ecstasy, and freedom. Entheogens are sacred visionary plant medicines that bring one into communion with Infinite Intelligence and plant, animal, and other intelligences who help us to broaden our understanding of ourselves, our purpose, and the nature of reality. Use of entheogens is an ancient practice that has healed, sourced, inspired, guided, and evolved human beings for eons. All ancient cultures have evolved with the guidance of sacred plant medicines, which have always taught humans the right way to live.

[10] Iatrogenic illnesses are caused by medical malpractice and medical interventions, procedures, drugs, and treatments often during hospital stays.

[11] The Fertility Crisis includes worldwide decreasing birthrates, declining fertility rates, increasing miscarriages and stillbirths, increasing genital abnormalities, lower sperm counts, reduced testosterone levels, and increasing gender dysphoria.

[12] Adrenochrome is produced by the body as a result of prolonged stress and pain. It is prized and harvested by the parasites for its euphoric, rejuvenating, and empowering properties.

Normalization of pedophilia and gender dysphoria. The Transgender Agenda. The Androgyny Agenda. Politicization and public sacrifice of children. The Troubled Teen industry. The youth suicide epidemic. Unacceptable incarceration rates. The prison business. Urban decay. The homelessness epidemic. The loneliness epidemic. Weaponized immigration.

The insidious and relentless dissemination of lies and misinformation through all sources. Digital dementia. Cyberwarfare. Cybercrimes. Mass public, personal, and online surveillance. Loss of personal freedom and human rights. Total dependence on government. The technocratic takeover. Democide. The depopulation agenda. Transhumanism. Consciousness Transfer technologies. The digital gulag. The rise of the Fourth Reich. The Nazification of our reality.

There is mounting evidence of crimes against Humanity, treason, terrorism, and systemic satanic ritual abuse being perpetrated within the echelons of power. Most people unknowingly participate in satanic rituals, including mass public humiliation rituals – mask-wearing; taking the knee; panic buying of toilet paper; skull, oral, and anal swabs; medical rape; and showing cards/chips/marks to prove obedience. Add to that live and televised satanic rituals, music concerts, music videos, entertainment industry award ceremonies, opening ceremonies for global sporting events and public infrastructure, half-time sports entertainment, and endless bombardment from advertising/brands/logos. Continuous public sacrificial and bloodletting rituals are now part of daily life – wars, genocides, the endless slaughter of animals for meat, cesarean deliveries, cutting umbilical cords, circumcisions, and abortions – all evidence of the presence of a satanic blood cult.

The fact is that almost every human being is terrorized, self-suffocating when wearing a mask,[13] imprisoned, depressed, confused, traumatized, suffering from PTSD, living life through a screen, and disconnected from Nature, from friends, from community, and from God.

What else explains the presence of such unthinkable and unspeakable Evil?

What explains the evidence and prevalence of all that is abhorrent and harmful to our species and hostile to the nature of the soul?

And how else to explain the endless saga of human misery and the global pandemic of suffering that only worsens?

What drives greed, selfishness, narcissism, and insatiable hunger for material possessions, sense gratification, and attention?

What is feeding the miasma of beastliness into innocent minds?

Why are there relentless assaults upon our inalienable right to be human – to live peacefully, in harmony with each other and with Nature, to make our own choices about our health, our livelihood, our movements, our family life, and our social life?

What is driving the technocratic tranhumanist tyranny and the pharmaceutical biofascism takeover?

What else explains the war on joy, the war on community,,

---

[13] To breathe one's own breath repeatedly is to die.

and the war upon our ability to be healthy, to be happy, to be free, and to enjoy life?

Being in the wrong place at the wrong time?

Bad luck?

It is more like bad management.

Human nature, which is pure, Divine nature – to love, care for, help, and uplift all – is being hijacked and perverted by a malevolent, highly-evolved lifeform that understands human psychology far better than most humans. Humans are being defiled, debilitated, denatured, and devolved into a pathological, omnicidal species, devoid of empathy, common sense, courage, and spirituality, and our environment is reflecting the almost complete aberration and devolution of human nature.

Consciousness is the ability to perceive self and decode Life through the five physical senses and extrasensory perceptions. Our ability to perceive and decode reality and to make sense of what is going on in the world is being thwarted, polluted, and held within a narrow bandwidth by Masters of Mindfuckery using multiple strategies previously listed and others we may never know about.

***Light is the information of Truth.***
***Your ignorance is their power.***
***Knowledge is your power.***

At best, most humans are only able to perceive a microfraction of a fractal of reality. We see less than one percent of the visible light spectrum. Beyond the range of one's perception, there is an endlessly bigger picture. As we heal emotional wounds, expand consciousness, align free will with Divine Will, and evolve at a soul level, our ability to perceive more of reality expands. One of the many ways human beings have been disempowered, manipulated, and controlled is by preventing the expansion of human consciousness, which limits the ability to perceive a bigger picture and the true nature of reality, and prevents a connection with All That Is, access to higher knowledge, and activation of supersensory gifts and infinite power. Narrative warfare, Cognitive warfare, and NeuroPsychoCyber warfare are used to control the flow of information, which controls human behavior, and that is how the enslavement of humankind in an inverted, perverted, soul-sucking, false-reality mind matrix is achieved. These Demons of Deception then harness and direct human consciousness to generate low vibrational energy, to create hell on Earth, and to keep humans orchestrating, supporting, demanding, defending, and loving the systems of their own enslavement. It's evil genius.

> **"The ability to hold Light is directly proportional to the courage to see Darkness."**
> – GALACTIC FEDERATION OF LIGHT

There are countless evil strategies being deployed to keep humans ignorant and enslaved, which is a testament to how powerful, priceless, and prized we are. Humankind is also under attack through physical warfare – poisoned food, water, and air supplies; highly processed foods; junk and fast foods; alcohol; pharmaceutical drugs; recreational drugs;

vaccinations/bioweapons; geoengineering; weaponization of our environment by chemicals, electromagnetism, and nanotechnologies; biowarfare; chemtrails; electromagnetic pollution; and frequency manipulations, which intentionally cause physical illnesses, severe brain damage, genetic modification, and pain and suffering. Brain-damaging chemicals (neurotoxins) are added to air, food, water, drugs, vaccines, and personal care and household products.[14] Detoxifying, decalcifying, protecting, and fueling the brain are essential practices to optimize personal power. Without optimal brain health, optimal health and well-being and spiritual evolution are not possible. One is rudderless, unable to connect with Infinite Intelligence, access Infinite Power, or discover Truth.

> ***Never be afraid of the Truth,***
> ***because the Truth will set us free.***
> ***Truth is power. Truth is the armor of God.***
> ***Ignore the Truth at your own peril,***
> ***and at the peril of our species.***

The truth is not always easy, pretty, or comfortable. The truth is sometimes ugly, brutal, shocking, terrifying, unimaginable, unfathomable, and unbearable. Most people would rather suffer and die than look within or realize the

---

[14] There are neurotoxins, carcinogens, and hormone disrupters in toothpaste, mouthwash, soaps, bodywash, shampoo, conditioner, sunscreen, makeup, nail polish and remover, hand sanitizers, hair dyes, perfumes, deodorants, artificial fragrances, air fresheners, laundry detergents, fabric softeners, dryer sheets, clothing, cleaning products, pesticides, public water supplies, highly processed foods, and chemtrails. Choose organic and natural alternatives.

Truth. The truth is that blind belief in authority is the greatest enemy of Truth. The truth is that those in power lie, and they continue to lie to stay in power. We have been lied to about who we are and why we are here. We have been lied to about our history, current events, and our future. The truth is that we have been lied to about almost everything, and we must unlearn all that we have learned. This synthetic, earthly reality matrix is deeply deceptive, and humankind has been duped into self-imposed slavery. Our organic reality and our organic timeline have been hijacked. A satanic inversion principle is in effect - good is evil and evil is good. Our true identity has been hidden, and essential information about the nature of reality and spirituality has been occulted (hidden).

> *"We are not human beings having  
> a spiritual experience.  
> We are spiritual beings having  
> a human experience."*  
> – Pierre Teilhard de Chardin

The truth is that we are Divine in nature. Each of us is an immortal, spiritual being of infinite Love/Light with infinite creative power and potential, and we are here in Earth School for the spiritualization of our soul. We are here to evolve. We are here live as multidimensional, sovereign beings in harmony with others and the Earth; to learn about emotions, limitation, and creation; to embody, radiate, and expand Love; to enrich our inner life; to create beauty; to contribute to the common good and the upliftment of others; and to enjoy life. We are here to remember and realign with our true nature, our Divine nature, and to ongoingly refine our nature. We are here to manifest our light body and shine with the light of a billion suns. We are not here to live as a food supply or as slaves for regressive, psychopathic life forms. We are not here to live in fear, to suffer, to follow cradle-to-grave scripts, to work to earn money to live, to be a debt slave, to amass material wealth, to accumulate material objects, to pay taxes that fund wars and unspeakable crimes, to follow immoral and unjust laws, to be poisoned, to support systems of control and perpetuate the tyranny of evil, or to destroy our home and the future of our children. We are not here to wait to be given permission to live as freeborn, sovereign, magnificent, Divine beings.

***Freedom and power come with the remembrance of oneself as Divine in nature.***

Besides a miracle and/or Divine Intervention, the solution to our predicament is for each of us to remember who we are and know the truth about where we come from, why we are here, and the enslavement of our species in order to understand what is really going on and what needs to change. If we do this, we can change course, both individually and collectively. We have infinite power to transform the world around us by first changing ourselves – from ignorant to informed; from weak to strong; from sick to thriving; from fearful to empowered; from selfish to selfless; from enslaved to sovereign; and from separated to unified with All That Is.

### *Now is the Kairos moment for Humanity.*

Now is our opportunity to take control and change course. Now is the time to choose between truth and lies, wisdom and ignorance, health and sickness, courage and cowardice, power and learned helplessness, Love and fear, and freedom and slavery. The global 'plandemic' has given us an extraordinary opportunity to pause, be still, ask questions, research, contemplate, meditate, and discover the Truth. A miraculous window of opportunity has been opened for all to recognize the war on humans, the predation upon Humanity, the hijacking of reality through perception deception, the intentional devolution of humankind, and the destruction of our ecosystem. With this knowledge, one can undo cult programming, break free from the mind prison and the technocratic web, prevent the evil endgame of the predators, restore our organic, Divine timeline, and co-create New Earth. This window of opportunity will close. It will not wait for you. Do not turn your back on this moment because it is a gift that will not come again. We are the last hope for our species, and unless we unite and fight for our rights and freedom, we are doomed.

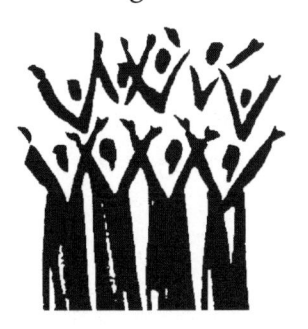

> *"A ruthless redemptive process must begin immediately within each of us, our communities, and all Nations."*
> – PHILLIP LINDSAY[15]

---

[15] www.esotericastrologer.org

To avoid the dystopian nightmare that the parasites intend for Humanity,[16] each of us must seize this opportunity and take immediate action to emancipate ourselves from mental slavery so we can come together in unity consciousness, with hearts radiating pure Love, to create a love-based reality, and enjoy life as sovereign beings living in harmony with each other, Nature, and with All That Is. To live as a sovereign being, one must become empowered and informed, which is not easy in this age of deception. One must become intolerant of all compromises to Truth, Natural Law, and freedom, and be peacefully non-compliant to all systems of control that are encroaching every day. Practice peaceful dissent. There are not enough police, military personnel, or prisons to contain all of us who offer unbreakable resistance and refuse to comply, take the jabs, or pay fines.

*"Alas, mental slavery is the worst form of slavery. It gives one the illusion of freedom, makes one trust, love, and defend one's oppressor, while making an enemy of those who are trying to free you, and to open your eyes!"*
– RICHARD C. IRITANO

*"When tyranny becomes law, rebellion becomes duty."*
– THOMAS JEFFERSON

---

[16] See the "*2030 Agenda for Sustainable Development*" from the playbook of the Chinese Communist Party ratified by the United Nations.: https://sdgs.un.org/2030agenda

Exactly how and why events are unfolding on the world stage is open for speculation, but the facts are not. Tragically, people are suffering and dying from "a virus called COVID-19" by governments, scientists, doctors, celebrities, and billionaire eugenicists and endlessly repeated by lying puppets and paid bad actors in the mainstream media/government propaganda machine. Under the guise of protecting public health and safety, Humanity is being subject to communist tactics, fear-based mind control, relentless propaganda, televised theatrics and spellcraft, Scientism, mindfuckery, numberfuckery, gaslighting, mockery, and relentless lies that are brainwashing and bamboozling humankind with the CV narrative and perpetuating the greatest lie ever told. There is a global psyop in effect. There is no fatal virus wiping out most of humankind, and thus no justification for locking down, suffocating, terrorizing, violating, vaccinating, and impoverishing most human beings for years with no end in sight. Recovery rates are over 99% for all age groups. Natural cures are effective.[17] Pharmaceuticals are effective.[18] Less than 1% of the world's population has died from COVID-19.[19] The majority of people

---

[17] Rona, Z. *Coronavirus Protection and Treatment: Top 10 Natural Remedies.* www.vitalitymagazine.com 15 October 2021
https://vitalitymagazine.com/article/coronavirus-protection-and-treatment-top-10-natural-remedies/

[18] Zelenko Protocols against Covid-19
https://vladimirzelenkomd.com/treatment-protocol/

[19] Bitchute: Emergency Broadcast - with guest Dr Ardis. therevealreport. 12 October 2021.
https://rumble.com/vnmmjr-emergency-broadcast-with-guest-dr-ardis.html

whose deaths were officially attributed to COVID-19 were elderly with comorbidity factors – immune-compromised. poisoned, and depleted from living in this toxic world that makes humans weak and vulnerable to illness and disease. There were no massive spikes in worldwide death rates from start of the plandemic in early 2020 until the injection experiment began.[20]

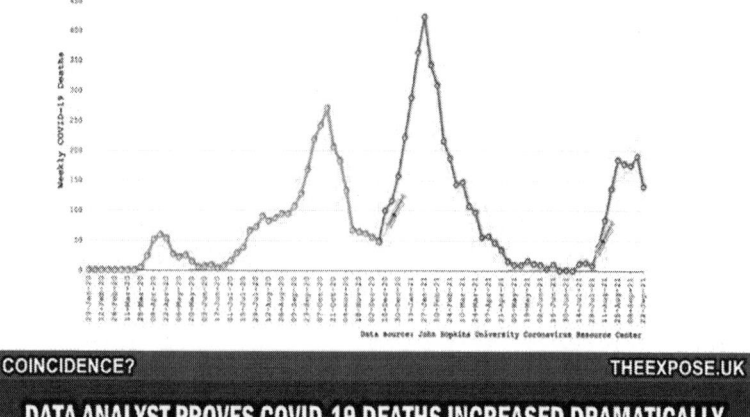

**COINCIDENCE?**             **THEEXPOSE.UK**

**DATA ANALYST PROVES COVID-19 DEATHS INCREASED DRAMATICALLY AFTER THE VACCINE ROLL-OUT IN OVER 40 COUNTRIES**

Hospitals, doctors, and medical staff are under orders perpetuate the pandemic lie one variant/scariant after another, to fill COVID wards, maximize profits for Big Pharma, and implement end-of-life protocols where possible. Doctors with integrity and courage are risking their lives and their livelihoods to speak out about what they are witnessing.

---

[20] The Expose. *Data Analyst proves Covid-19 Deaths increased dramatically AFTER the Vaccine roll-out in over 40 countries.* www.theexpose.uk 18 October 2021 https://theexpose.uk/2021/10/18/covid-19-deaths-increased-dramatically-after-the-vaccine-roll-out-in-over-40-countries/

Patients are dying with CV, not from CV, as a result of hospital protocols and jab injuries. They are reporting that CV death tolls are grossly overinflated because deaths from adverse reactions to the shots and other pre-existing conditions are included in the statistics.[21] The majority of COVID hospitalizations and deaths are fully vaccinated people.[22] Many physicians have stated that there is, in fact, no deadly virus pandemic at all and no basis for declaring and perpetuating a state of emergency.[23] There is the official narrative, there are bioweapons, and there is the sinister truth. A seasonal respiratory virus of high infectivity and low pathogenicity is being used as a Trojan horse to usher in a New World Order. There is a well-planned, socially engineered, perceived crisis, which is being leveraged to generate terror, trauma,

---

[21] Rumble: ATTORNEY THOMAS RENZ "We Got Them. Fact Check This!" ALL NEW WHISTLEBLOWER INFO. BookitCJ. 27 September 2021 https://rumble.com/vn12v1-attorney-thomas-renz-we-got-them.-fact-check-this-all-new-whistleblower-inf.html

[22] TLB Staff. *89% of COVID-19 Deaths Among Fully Vaccinated*. www.europereloaded.com.au. 25 November 2021. https://www.europereloaded.com/89-of-covid-19-deaths-among-the-fully-vaccinated-latest-data/

[23] Doctors speaking out about the COVID-19 psyop and the extreme dangers of the COVID-19 injection are being censored on all platforms. If one person is not free to speak, no-one is free to speak. Censorship is the enemy of freedom.
Millions Against Medical Mandates: https://mamm.org/
 Doctors for Covid Ethics: https://doctors4covidethics.org/
World Doctors Alliance: https://worlddoctorsalliance.com/
Americas Frontline Doctors: https://www.americasfrontlinedoctors.org/
PANDA (Pandemics Data Analysis): https://www.pandata.org/team/
FLCCC Alliance (Front Line COVID-19 Critical Care Alliance); https://covid19criticalcare.com/
HART (Health Advisory and Recovery Team): https://www.hartgroup.org/
Children's Health Defense Fund. https://childrenshealthdefense.org/
Covid Medical Network: https://www.covidmedicalnetwork.com/

cowardice, inaction, mistrust, division, and submission; to strip human rights and freedom through draconian measures; and to establish centralized government, totalitarianism, and the total enslavement of humankind.[24]

COVID-19 is the flu rebranded and weaponized to provide a smokescreen and a distraction. All mandates, rules, bills, policies, and "laws" that are implemented worldwide to "control a deadly virus" have nothing to do with preventing deaths, protecting us, improving health and safety, or with a virus or virology. These measures are being implemented to destroy our health, our personal power, our livelihoods, our communities, our families, our freedom, and our future. All government and corporate public health strategies disempower and weaken us, individually and collectively, while transferring incalculable wealth and power to a small number of despicable lowlifes with purely selfish and satanic intentions. We are witnessing the greatest episode of internal looting ever recorded. Continuing to believe in the false narrative of a global virus pandemic - the Great Deception - is one of the most disempowering choices an individual can make at this time.

*They lied about THALIDOMIDE. They lied about ASBESTOS. They lied about CIGARETTES. They lied about FLOURIDE in drinking water and toothpaste. They lied about SATURATED*

---

[24] See Event 201, 18 October 2019. New York, USA: https://www.centerforhealthsecurity.org/event201/]

*FATS, ANIMAL PROTEIN,* and *DAIRY MILK. They lied about ALCOHOL, SUGAR, HIGH FRUCTOSE CORN SYRUP,* and *ARTIFICIAL SWEETENERS. They lied about MERCURY FILLINGS. They lied about ALUMINIUM in deodorants. They lied about TALC in hygiene products. They lied about LEAD in paint. They lied about CHEMOTHERAPY and RADIATION. They lied about CHOLESTEROL and STATIN drugs. They lied about HORMONE REPLACEMENT THERAPY. They lied about the safety of PHARMACEUTICAL DRUGS, OPIODS, and VACCINES. They lied about PESTCIDES, ROUNDUP, DDT, and GLYPHOSATE. They lied about GMOs, CARCINOGENIC FOODS, and FAST FOODS. They lie about OVERPOPULATION and EXTRATERRESTRIALS. They lie about CLIMATE CHANGE. They are lying about EMFs and 5G. They are lying about a VIRUS PANDEMIC and ASYMPTOMATIC TRANSMISSION. They are lying about IMMUNITY-DESTROYING, GENE-ALTERING, MIND-CONTROLLING INJECTIBLES. They are lying about their TRUE AGENGA, which is to arrest the earthy development of humans, impose a synthetic, soulless, transhuman timeline for Humanity, and usher in another GREAT RESET.*

If any government genuinely cared about the health and well-being of its citizens, there would be action taken to address, treat, curb, and prevent easily preventable deaths[25] from the biggest killers of humans – heart disease and cancer, which remain the biggest killers of human beings after 2 years of the scamdemic.[26] But instead of taking any effective actions to prevent millions of deaths annually, governments, in collaboration with drug and chemical companies and other perpetrators of evil upon humankind, subsidize the production and distribution of foods and beverages that cause heart disease and cancers. And they peddle pharmaceutical drugs as cures that instead create more suffering, cause early deaths, and generate egregious profits.

> *"A patient cured is a customer lost."*
> – BIG PHARMA

Governments are nefarious webs of maleficence that control, tax/milk/steal from, weaken, and sicken people in order to accumulate greater power and wealth for the obscenely powerful and wealthy. Governments give people the illusion of safety and security, but governments are criminal gangs of Satanists, psychopaths, sociopaths,

---

[25] Eating nutritious, natural foods, regular exercise, stress reduction, and spending time in Nature helps to prevent heart disease and cancers.

[26] Chander, V. *COVID-19 third leading cause of U.S. deaths in 2020 after heart disease, cancer: U.S. report.* www.reuters.com 31 March 2021. https://www.reuters.cMm/article/us-health-coronavirus-usa-mortality/covid-19-third-leading-cause-of-u-s-deaths-in-2020-after-heart-disease-cancer-u-s-report-idUSKBN2BN2KD?edition-redirect=in

pedophiles, and paid liars who profit at our expense and make life worse for all of us at every opportunity. Governments are in place to create dependency; to keep us fearful, sick, powerless, impoverished, and living as slaves for oligarchs; and to continuously interfere with our lives and our livelihoods to prevent us from enjoying life and liberty. Believing that governments serve the people is one of the most disempowering beliefs one can cling to. Continuing to trust in Government is naïve and dangerous. The system is corrupt to its core. False beliefs and misplaced trust in governments are the reasons almost the entire human population is terrified, muzzled, under house arrest due to COVID-19, jobless, hopeless, exasperated, suffering from PTSD, and poisoned with untested, life-threatening, gene-altering,[27] sterilizing, zombifying experimental injectables.

***"The conscious and intelligent manipulation of the organized habits and opinions of the masses is an important element in a democratic society. Those who manipulate this unseen mechanism***

---

[27] Legally, jabs recipients are no longer human. In a 2013 court case, Association for Molecular Pathology et. al. v Myriad Genetics, Inc., the US Supreme Court ruled that human DNA could not be patented, because it is 'a product of nature.' The Supreme Court ruled that if a human genome is modified by mRNA vaccines (which are currently in use), then the genome can be patented. All jab recipients are now technically 'patented,' and something that is patented is 'proprietary' and will be included in the definition of 'transhuman.' People who are legally identified as 'transhuman' do not have access to human rights or rights granted by the state because they are no longer classified as 100% biological or human. They are GMOs.
https://www.supremecourt.gov/opinions/12pdf/12-398_1b7d.pdf

> ***of society constitute an invisible government, which is the true ruling power of our country."***
> – EDWARD BERNAYS

Courage is the armor of God. It takes great courage to face the truth that humankind is enslaved, government is slavery, and the solution is not political. Emancipation from mental slavery through a revolution of consciousness is the solution. Anarchy is the answer – living in alignment with Cosmic Spiritual Law under self-governance with no masters and no slaves. It takes great courage, effort, and personal sacrifice to embody freedom, align with Truth, and become fully empowered. One must be willing to trust, surrender, and go through the eye of the needle at least once.

We have unlimited power to create, the power to destroy, and the power to control ourselves and others. We have the power to choose, the power to change, and the power to protect and defend ourselves and others from danger. We have the power to unlock our full potential and change the world. We have powers that have yet to be revealed. We can use our power for whatever we choose: for good and for evil; to heal and to harm; and for selfless and selfish reasons.

### *Selfishness is the root of all evil.*

Most people want power to control life, to get what they want (money, sex, possessions, attention, reputation, relationships), and/or to control other people and life events, but using personal power in any of these ways is wrong and leads to suffering and loss of true power. Scheming, scamming, deceiving, and manipulating others dissipates energy and destroys physical and mental health. Using personal power for purely self-serving reasons is evil and strengthens the presence of evil within self and within this reality. Using personal power to get what one wants may bring material and transitory sensorial results, but the overall result will be a life lived in service to self, which is the definition of evil. Schools of Thought, "spiritual teachers," New Thought leaders, religious leaders, and Influencers who encourage the use of personal power for personal gain without considering the common good are inherently evil.[28]

This deception in the New Age movement is diabolical and begins with the desecration of Natural Law. Case in point: The Law of Attraction/Vibration has been taken out of context and sold as *"The Secret."* This is an excellent example of how individual power is manipulated to serve self/Evil. Instead of being introduced to Natural Law (which is the highest Truth), spiritual seekers in the New Age movement have been presented with only one Principle, when actually

---

[28] The New Age movement is another psyop. Followers are duped into serving Evil by the notion that not paying attention to Evil in this world and/or not believing that Evil exists will either make Evil go away, or not exist at all. But ignoring the presence, power, and scope of Evil allows Evil to flourish. Facing Evil within self, and in the world, is a necessary step to ending suffering, violence, wars, environmental destruction, child abuse, slavery, addictions, and destruction of our ecosystem. The grip of religions (including the New Age movement, Government, and Money) upon most of the human population is firm but waning, because the vibrational frequency of Earth is that of Love, and all systems that control humans that are fear-based and lacking integrity, accountability, transparency, equality, and Truth are no longer sustainable.

there are seven: Mentalism, Correspondence, Attraction/Vibration, Polarity, Rhythm, Causality, and Gender. Yet only the Law of Attraction/Vibration is peddled as *"The Secret"* and touted as the way to get what you want, rather than the way to serve the highest good of all. Without knowledge of all seven principles,[29] an individual is ignorant of Cosmic Spiritual Law (the *real* secret), and thus disempowered, unbalanced, and ultimately serving self/Evil.

True power is freedom from self-limitations, fears, emotional wounds, false beliefs, limiting subconscious programming, addictions, delusions, deceptions, and from inner poverty – loss of connection to All That Is. True power is self-awareness, self-correction, self-confidence, self-love, and self-mastery. True power means control over self. Those who pursue material wealth, fame, and power over others will be destroyed by their own ambition.

> ***"The power is within you. It always has been. How far are you willing to expand the horizons of your thinking and stir that power awake?"***
> – Louise Hay[30]

True power means control over self (emotions, speech, behaviors, and needs) and never control over others. True power is freedom from the dominance of others, from man-made policies, possessions, and the illusory structures of

---

[29] See *Natural Law* on page 40..

[30] www.hayhouse.com

time and space. True power gives access to and control of limitless inner resources. True power is infinite good and infinite Love. True power is the armor of God.

***Invoke and embody the power of
Infinite Intelligence and the forces of Light
at every opportunity.***

With great power comes great responsibility. If an individual does not take responsibility for personal power by harnessing it to serve the common good, it will be squandered and/or vampirized by other people and malevolent life forms and used for their sustenance and empowerment. Taking full responsibility for one's personal power and using it to serve the highest good of all is the optimal use of personal power and the only way to create health, happiness, harmony, and peace on Earth.

Free will cannot be violated unless permission/consent is given. Compliance, nonresistance, silence, and voting give consent to being ruled.

***"Qui tacet consentit" is translated as "Silence
gives consent." This is why "silence is golden."
Our silence gives the false gods a claim on our
created elixir of immortality – Golden blood
plasma – the ether of the heart."***
— Chiron Last[31]

---

[31] YouTube: *The House of EL*. Chiron Last. 8 June 2015.

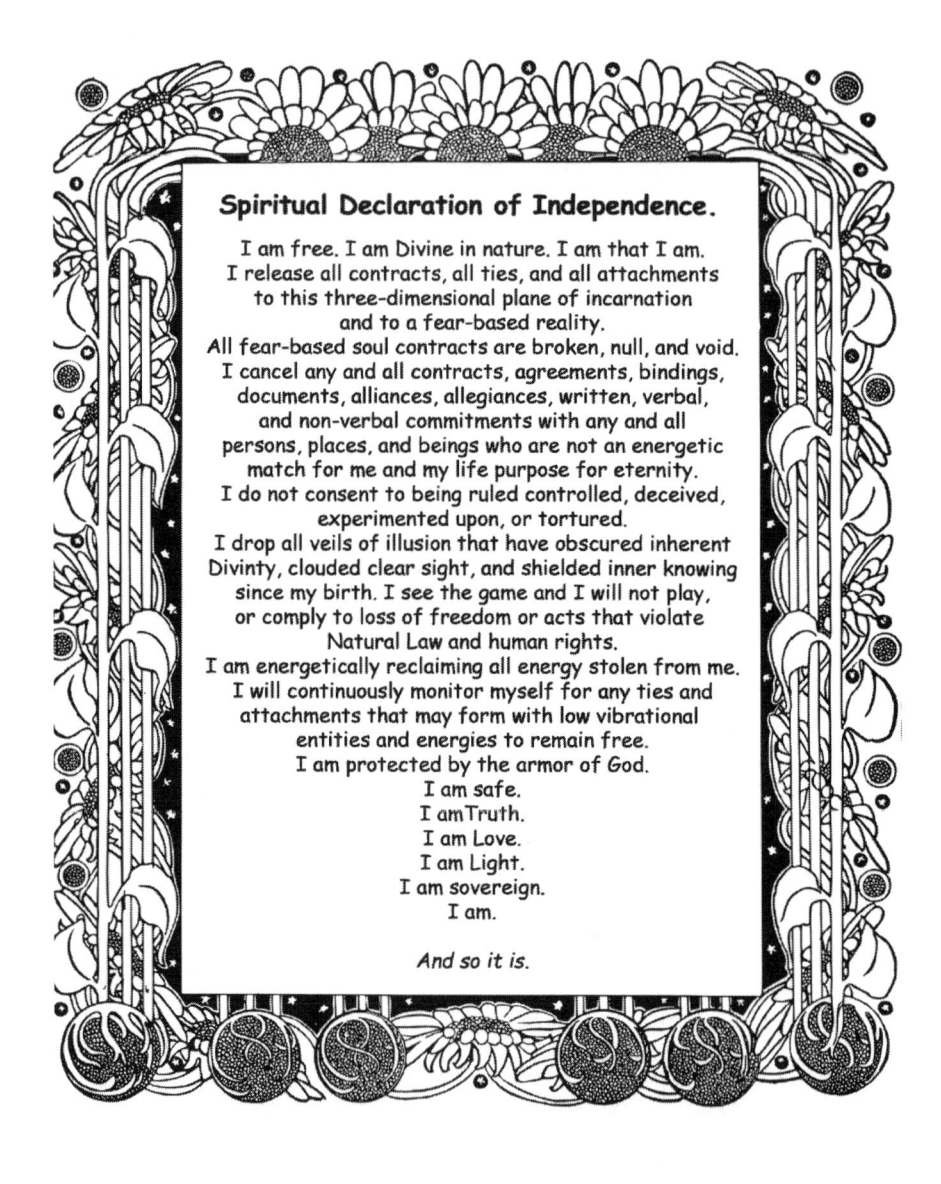

## Spiritual Declaration of Independence.

I am free. I am Divine in nature. I am that I am.
I release all contracts, all ties, and all attachments
to this three-dimensional plane of incarnation
and to a fear-based reality.
All fear-based soul contracts are broken, null, and void.
I cancel any and all contracts, agreements, bindings,
documents, alliances, allegiances, written, verbal,
and non-verbal commitments with any and all
persons, places, and beings who are not an energetic
match for me and my life purpose for eternity.
I do not consent to being ruled controlled, deceived,
experimented upon, or tortured.
I drop all veils of illusion that have obscured inherent
Divinity, clouded clear sight, and shielded inner knowing
since my birth. I see the game and I will not play,
or comply to loss of freedom or acts that violate
Natural Law and human rights.
I am energetically reclaiming all energy stolen from me.
I will continuously monitor myself for any ties and
attachments that may form with low vibrational
entities and energies to remain free.
I am protected by the armor of God.
I am safe.
I amTruth.
I am Love.
I am Light.
I am sovereign.
I am.

*And so it is.*

Immediately revoke all agreements with forces of evil. Declare all soul contracts with dark forces null and void. Make a Declaration of Sovereignty and establish permanent protection.[32] Claim independence from all evil entities and social systems of control. Do not consent to experiences of suffering, to external rulership, or to soul traps. Declare freedom from all soul traps and Earth recycling traps for this life and beyond. There are many layers to these soul agreements, so it is beneficial to ongoingly reaffirm non-consent to external rulership throughout all time and space, to practice peaceful non-compliance to tyranny, and to align with peace, love, truth, beauty, and joy. There is nothing to fear. Only Love is real.

> *There are only two paths to follow.*
> *One leads to increased health, happiness, power, and freedom.*
> *The other path leads to increased ill-health, weakness, fear, suffering, and enslavement.*
> *The choice is yours in every moment.*

Increased personal power comes though understanding human nature, Divine nature, Nature, and Natural Law. Optimal personal power comes through living in balance and in alignment with Natural Law, with Cosmic Spiritual

---

https://www.youtube.com/watch?v=oxTP6wLxQxo&feature=youtu.be

[32] See opposite page for an example of a Spiritual Declaration of Independence: Writing and stating aloud your own declaration is most empowering.

with the 42 Ideals of Ma'at[33], and with one's rsonal power consists of spiritual power, mental ower, the power of speech, physical power, sexual power, financial power, and our collective power. We have the power of intention, the power of desire, and the power of choice. We are omnipotent.

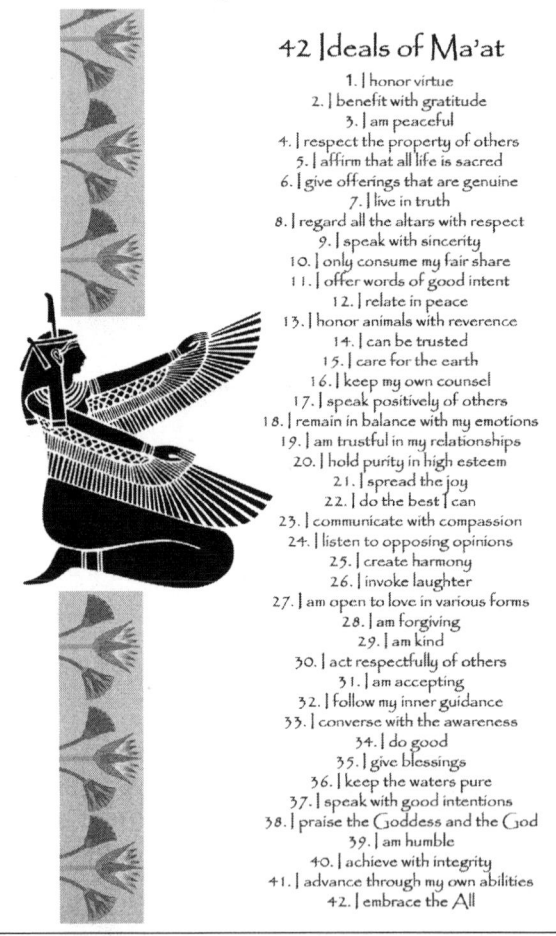

### 42 Ideals of Ma'at

1. I honor virtue
2. I benefit with gratitude
3. I am peaceful
4. I respect the property of others
5. I affirm that all life is sacred
6. I give offerings that are genuine
7. I live in truth
8. I regard all the altars with respect
9. I speak with sincerity
10. I only consume my fair share
11. I offer words of good intent
12. I relate in peace
13. I honor animals with reverence
14. I can be trusted
15. I care for the earth
16. I keep my own counsel
17. I speak positively of others
18. I remain in balance with my emotions
19. I am trustful in my relationships
20. I hold purity in high esteem
21. I spread the joy
22. I do the best I can
23. I communicate with compassion
24. I listen to opposing opinions
25. I create harmony
26. I invoke laughter
27. I am open to love in various forms
28. I am forgiving
29. I am kind
30. I act respectfully of others
31. I am accepting
32. I follow my inner guidance
33. I converse with the awareness
34. I do good
35. I give blessings
36. I keep the waters pure
37. I speak with good intentions
38. I praise the Goddess and the God
39. I am humble
40. I achieve with integrity
41. I advance through my own abilities
42. I embrace the All

---

[33] To increase personal power, study, repeat, and uphold the 42 Ideals of Ma'at, the activating tenets of Natural Law and of Life. Ma'at is the Ancient Egyptian organizing principle of Truth, balance, order, harmony, Law, morality, justice, and Love.

# INCREASING SPIRITUAL POWER

*It is only when we realize our Oneness with Prime Creator that we become filled with its power.*

Spiritual power is the power that comes from within oneself – our quintessence. Spiritual power is also known as Divine power, Inner/Soul power, Metaphysical power, Psychotronic power, Lifeforce energy, Vital energy, Kundalini, Prana, Mana, Chi, Shakti, and Luminescence. Spiritual power is inherent and infinite. Spiritual power comes from a connection with self, Nature, and God. Spiritual power is the cumulative power generated by the unfoldment of our highest potential through spiritual practices, which accumulates in the mind as Light. Spiritual power is the essence of vitality within the body that strengthens immune function, healing, rejuvenation, resilience, courage, and perseverance. Spiritual power is the power of Love that radiates through the human heart, which can be increased by intention, attention, and acts of kindness, altruism, selfless service, and creativity. Love is the greatest power. Love is the power of healing, transformation, freedom, manifesting dreams, and miracles. Authentic Love and the authentic self are what remain after we heal emotional wounds and when we establish connection with the indwelling God. Love is the armor of God.

> *"The power you have is to be the best version of yourself you can be, so you can create a better world."*
> – Ashley Rickards

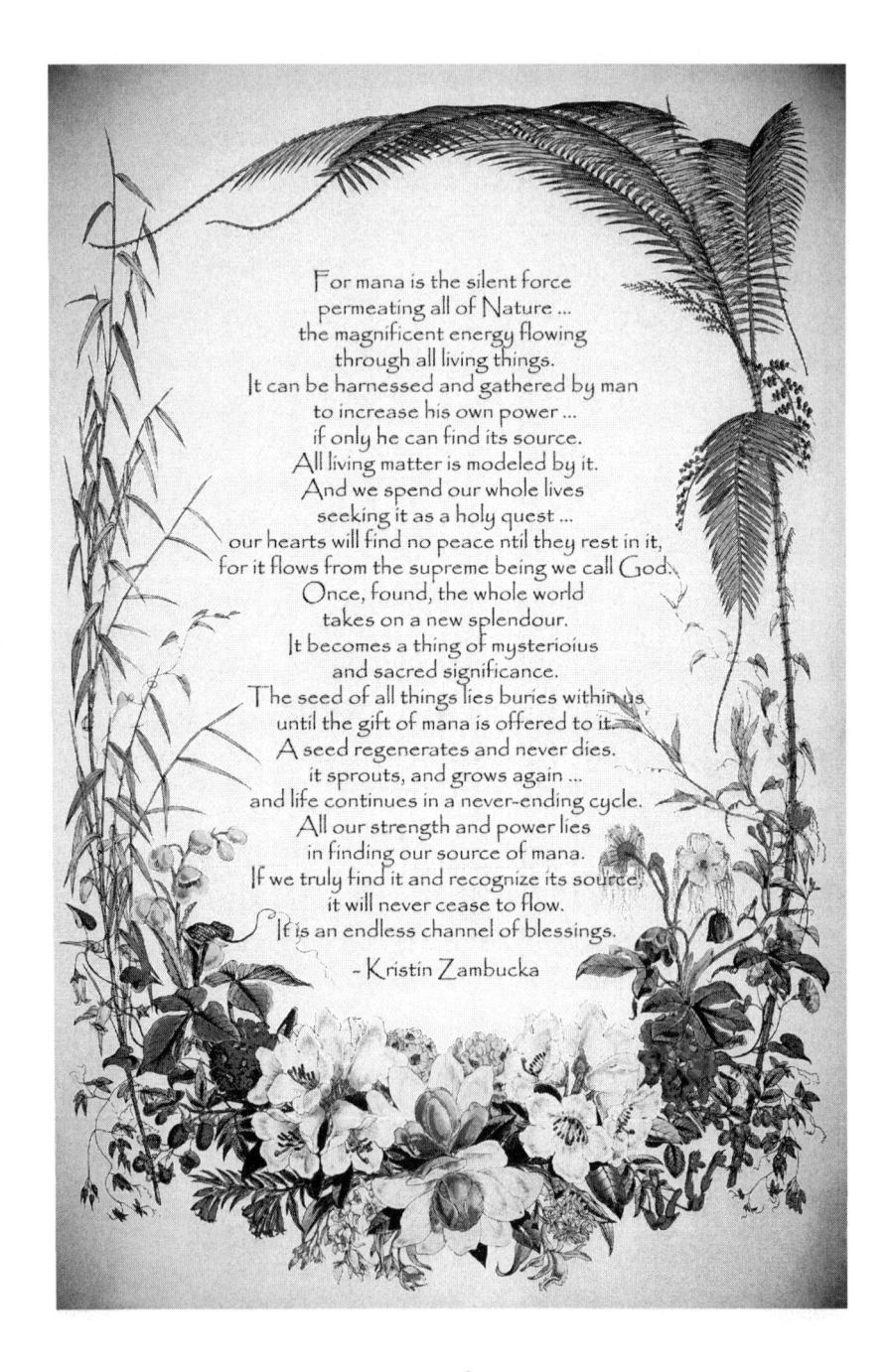

For mana is the silent force
permeating all of Nature ...
the magnificent energy flowing
through all living things.
It can be harnessed and gathered by man
to increase his own power ...
if only he can find its source.
All living matter is modeled by it.
And we spend our whole lives
seeking it as a holy quest ...
our hearts will find no peace ntil they rest in it,
for it flows from the supreme being we call God.
Once, found, the whole world
takes on a new splendour.
It becomes a thing of mysterioius
and sacred significance.
The seed of all things lies buries within us
until the gift of mana is offered to it.
A seed regenerates and never dies.
it sprouts, and grows again ...
and life continues in a never-ending cycle.
All our strength and power lies
in finding our source of mana.
If we truly find it and recognize its source,
it will never cease to flow.
It is an endless channel of blessings.

- Kristin Zambucka

> *"The more love you give in your day-to-day life, the greater the magnetic power of Love you have in the field around you, and everything you desire will fall at your feet."*
> — MAGDALENA HINCHCLIFFE

Spiritual power protects from evil and accumulates over lifetimes. Spiritual power can be harnessed and directed to serve the highest good of all, to heal oneself and others, and to change the nature of reality. The highest ideal for Humanity will be achieved through individual actualization of spiritual power, which is derived from following a spiritual path – serving God, doing inner work and spiritual practices with the intention of healing, expanding consciousness, embodying greater Love, and alchemizing the soul. Inner soul power comes with spiritual growth. One cannot expect Life to get better without becoming a better person.

> *"True knowledge can only come from the heart of an enlightened person."*
> — EVA WONG[34]

There are countless ancient wisdom traditions dedicated to increasing, harnessing, and directing spiritual power through spiritual practices, lifestyle practices, foods, herbs, and sacred plant medicines.

The following principles are shared by all ageless wisdom schools:

---
[34] www.limitlessgate.com

- There are as many paths as there are people.
- Desire to know and serve the Creator.
- Take every opportunity to deepen in relationship with God/Intelligent Infinity.
- Trust yourself. All that you need is found within.
- An intermediary between oneself and God is disempowering and unnecessary.
- Align Free Will with Divine Will.

*Let Thy will be my will.*
*Let Thy will be done through and unto me.*
*Thank You for the opportunity to serve*
*as an instrument of Divine Will.*

- Ask for and follow Divine guidance.
- Devote one's Life to seeking and serving Truth.
- Meditate daily. Make it a frequent practice to withdraw attention from the external, material world and pay attention to the inner, spiritual world.
- Study and live in accordance with Natural Law.

## NATURAL LAW

*"Natural Law is the body of existing, universal, eternal, inherent, objective, non-man-made, binding, and immutable conditions which act as the governing dynamics for consequences of behaviors of beings with the capacity for understanding the difference between harmful*

> *and non-harmful behavior.*
> *Natural Law is a body of universal Spiritual Laws, which act as the governing dynamics of Consciousness. Consciousness is the ability of a being to recognize patterns and meaning with respect to events taking place, both within oneself and in the realm in which the self exists and operates. It is our ability to perceive Truth.*
> *The understanding of Natural Law is centered upon the knowledge of Objective Morality and the alignment of our behavior to Objective Morality. This means we must know which behaviors are Rights because they do NOT initiate harm to other sentient beings, and which behaviors are Wrongs because they DO initiate harm to other sentient beings."*
> – Mark Passio[35]

Natural Law is immutable, ever-present, omnipresent, outside of space and time, and exists in the fabric of Life as the objective, inherent reality. Natural Law is not statutory law or man-made law and has nothing to do with any religion. Natural Law is Cosmic Spiritual Law. It is the underlying principle of the evolutionary process of Creation. It is the harmonizing and renewing force of the Cosmos. Natural Law is Truth, justice, freedom, harmony, balance, equality, and Love. Natural Law governs the consequences of human behavior. Like gravity and

---

[35] YouTube: *Mark Passio – The Deadly Pandemic That's Killing Anarchy*. Mark Passio. 10 May 2021. https://www.youtube.com/watch?v=lGUMFb9KZfs

electromagnetism, its existence and effects are not subject to or affected by beliefs or opinions. One cannot break Natural Law without suffering. One suffers as much from ignorant violations of Natural Law as from intentional violations.

> *"Most ailments begin with a corruption of Natural Law.*
> – MANLY P. HALL[36]

Understanding that there are Laws and principles inherent in Creation affecting all life throughout the Cosmos, life on Earth, and human consciousness and behavior is empowering. With knowledge, understanding, and application of Natural Law, one is empowered to create reality – heaven on Earth. Without knowledge or understanding of Natural Law, one is easily manipulated to create this earthly reality – hell on Earth. Without an understanding of Natural Law and the true nature of reality, humankind remains enslaved and suffering from mass hypnosis, mass delusion, and mass psychosis. Humanity is in a trance, and it is time for transcendence – the end of the trance – through knowledge of Natural Law.

> *"The purpose of reason is to become aware of the great rules, laws, and principles that sustain life."*
> – MANLY P. HALL[37]

---

[36] Hall, Manly. P. (1928). *The Secret Teachings of All Ages,* H.S. Crocker Company Inc., San Francisco. http://www.istitutocintamani.org/libri/The_secret_teachings_of_all_ages.pdf

[37] YouTube: *Organizing and Conserving Personal Energy Resources - Manly P. Hall*

Knowledge of Natural Law has been occulted in order to keep humans ignorant and powerless. A human who lives in accordance with Natural Law becomes balanced and divinely protected, divinely inspired, divinely guided, divinely empowered, and blessed beyond measure. Those who do not live in alignment with the principles of Natural Law, through ignorance or by choice, are unbalanced, powerless, and easily controlled and manipulated to serve evil agendas. Without knowledge of Universal Laws, no one and nothing can change for the better, and freedom is just a word. No good comes from ignoring Natural Law.

> *"Universal Law is the greatest good, the greatest beauty, the greatest Love, the greatest wisdom that man can know. Universal Law exists to permit and sustain the eternal unfoldment of life. This Law will preserve, perfect, and protect every creature that is true to it. Law finally becomes the blazing, living symbol of Divine Power, itself. Universal Law is Divine Will in operation."*
> — MANLY P. HALL[38]

It is in our best interest to understand and align with the principles of Natural Law. Living in harmony with Natural

---

*(Full Lecture/Clean Audio)*, MindPodNetwork. 8 July 2019. https://www.youtube.com/watch?v=A3aHeaODoJE

[38] YouTube: *The Seven Laws Governing Human Life by Manly P Hall*. Uncle Evey. 29 June 2019. https://www.youtube.com/watch?v=J2Pjze_UlZY&feature=youtu.be

Law means understanding and aligning with the universal principles in operation – the principles of Mentalism, Correspondence, Vibration, Polarity, Rhythm, Causality, and Gender, and the hidden, encapsulating principle of Care.[39]

### 7 Principles of Natural Law - Cosmic Spiritual Law

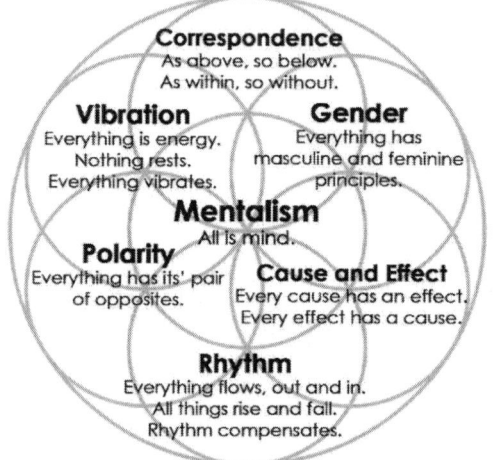

**Correspondence**
As above, so below.
As within, so without.

**Vibration**
Everything is energy.
Nothing rests.
Everything vibrates.

**Gender**
Everything has masculine and feminine principles.

**Mentalism**
All is mind.

**Polarity**
Everything has its' pair of opposites.

**Cause and Effect**
Every cause has an effect.
Every effect has a cause.

**Rhythm**
Everything flows, out and in.
All things rise and fall.
Rhythm compensates.

The **Principle of Care** encapsulates all other principles.
Care is the ultimate generative principle.

Living in harmony with Natural Law means living in balance and in alignment with Divine Will. Living in harmony with Natural Law means choosing to think, speak, and act in ways that do no harm to other lifeforms, and choosing morally right behavior over morally wrong/immoral behavior. Living in alignment with Natural Law means never infringing upon the free will of another lifeform. When in doubt as to whether

---

[39] YouTube: *Mark Passio & The Science Of Natural Law Documentary.* Mark Passio. 11 November 2021. https://www.youtube.com/watch?v=bP5sk5xp9WM&t=6s
Also on other platforms: www.whatonearthishappening.com and www.onegreatworknetwork.com.

any action is in harmony with Natural Law, it is necessary to assess if any harm is being done and if free will is being violated:

A morally right action is based in Truth, in harmony with Natural Law, and does not result in harm to another sentient being.

A morally wrong action is not based in Truth, not in harmony with Natural Law, and results in harm to another lifeform.

We have free will to choose how we live, but we are not free from the consequences of our choices because Natural Law is deterministic. Natural Law is a mirror. You reap what you sow. Every thought, word, action, and inaction has a consequence, and nobody is above the Law. We have free will and we are free to do whatever we choose, but we are not free from the consequences of our choices – our thoughts, words, and deeds. Freedom is not the ability to do whatever we want to do. It is the ability to align free will with Divine Will and do what is right, moral, and good for all of us, now and at least seven generations into the future. We derive power through knowledge and application of Natural Law. Ultimate power comes from alignment with what is right, true, and moral. Living in accordance with Natural Law creates order, balance, harmony, empowerment, prosperity, freedom, and sustainability. Living in ignorance of Natural Law, and not in accordance with its principles, creates chaos and imbalance, perpetuates suffering, and brings us closer to extinction. We have the right to use force in self-defense and to stop violations of Natural Law.

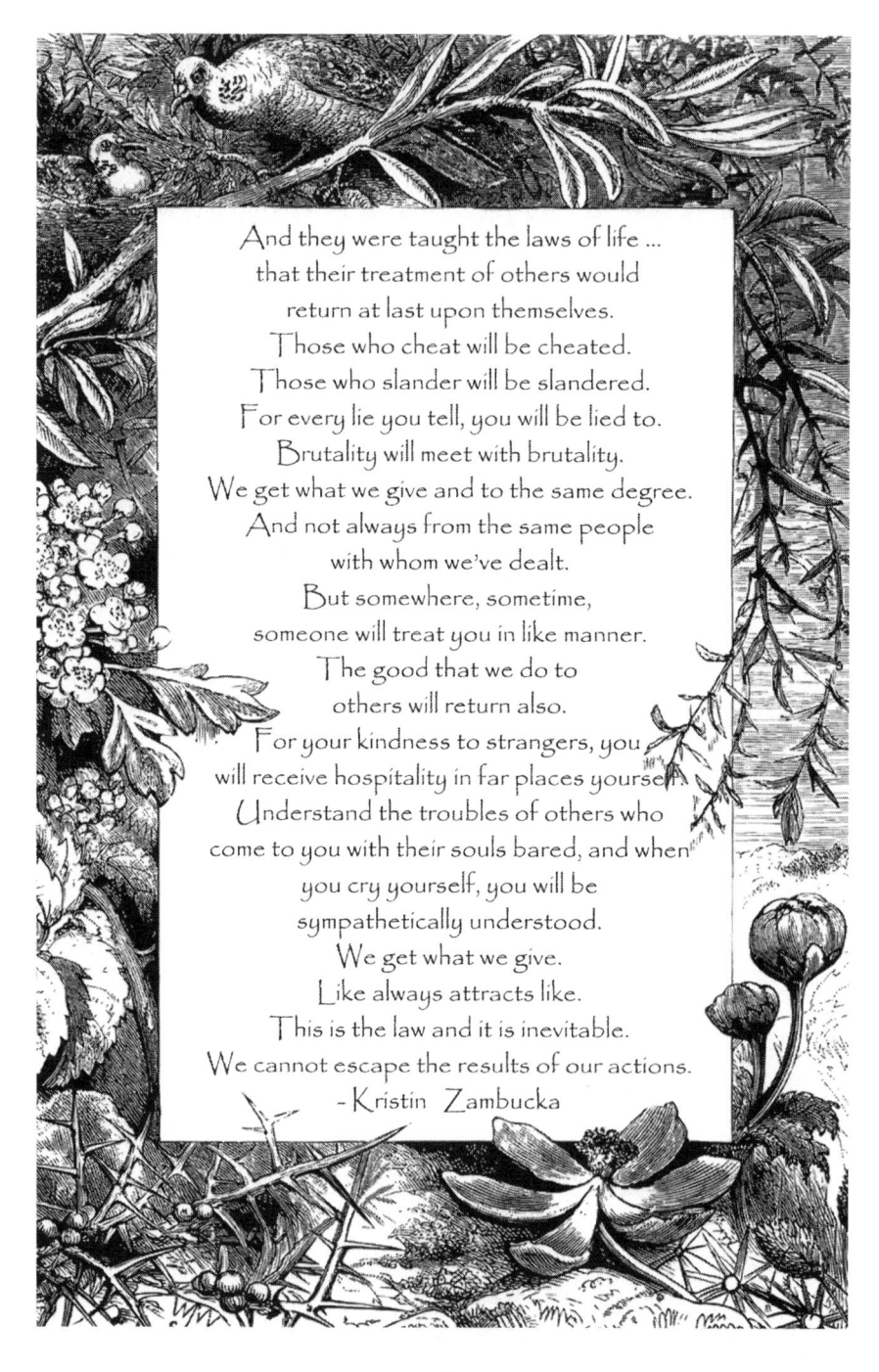

And they were taught the laws of life ...
that their treatment of others would
return at last upon themselves.
Those who cheat will be cheated.
Those who slander will be slandered.
For every lie you tell, you will be lied to.
Brutality will meet with brutality.
We get what we give and to the same degree.
And not always from the same people
with whom we've dealt.
But somewhere, sometime,
someone will treat you in like manner.
The good that we do to
others will return also.
For your kindness to strangers, you
will receive hospitality in far places yourself.
Understand the troubles of others who
come to you with their souls bared, and when
you cry yourself, you will be
sympathetically understood.
We get what we give.
Like always attracts like.
This is the law and it is inevitable.
We cannot escape the results of our actions.
     - Kristin Zambucka

*"Natural Law is the Law of Freedom.
Freedom and morality are directly proportional.
As morality increases, freedom increases.
As morality decreases, freedom decreases.
The presence of Truth and Morality in the lives
of the people of any given society is inversely
proportional to the presence of
Tyranny and Slavery in that society."*
– Mark Passio

Humanity is now suffering from the aggregate effects of violations against Natural Law from remote antiquity. Living in alignment with what is right, true, good, and moral will end suffering and confer limitless power. Only those who do no harm can be free. Only those who are engaged in right action evolve spiritually. Above all else, live by these principles, develop a moral compass, and pursue Truth, self-knowledge, and self-mastery. The future lies in the minds, hearts, and hands of those who live in alignment with Natural Law.

*"For only through Law comes the freedom of man."*
– Thoth

Know thyself. "Who am I?" is the most important question to ask and answer. Self-empowerment comes through knowledge about oneself, including one's Divine nature, ancestry, shadow side, and purpose. Self-knowledge is the source of greatest power. The more self-knowledge is acquired, the more empowered one becomes. Introspection, self-correction, and self-refinement build spiritual power.

Tools include Astrology,[40] Numerology, Alchemy, Human Design, I Ching, Tarot, Cards of the Illumination,[41] Channeling, Divination, The Seven Rays, Psychometric questionnaires, Personality Types, Enneagram, Journaling, Automatic Writing, Traveling, Meditation, Mental Health Therapy, a Master, a Mentor, a close friend, guides from other dimensions and timelines, and intuition.

Without some knowledge of Astrology and personal astrology, one is powerless and clueless. Our predators gain power from aligning their all plans and actions with empowering celestial events and alignments. Study Astrology for self-knowledge, self-betterment, and self-empowerment; to find purpose; to awaken super-genius; and for answers to any questions. Align actions, ventures, and adventures with moon cycles and planetary cycles for empowerment. Simple moon magic: New Moon energy supports new beginnings. Full Moon energy brings fruition. Use apps to track moon cycles and planetary positions.

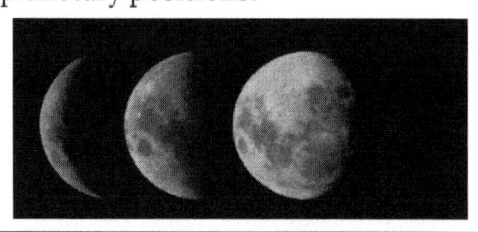

---

[40] The science of Astrology has been intentionally hijacked and confuscated to disempower us and deprive us of self-knowledge and universal knowledge, so choose an accurate system. Western Astrology is highly inaccurate. Sidereal Astrology is less inaccurate. We are all being double-crossed. Using the actual positions of celestial bodies via a program such as Stellarium (www.stellarium.org) is an accurate system.

[41] www.7thunders.com

Turn awareness inward and practice self-observation, self-analysis, and self-reflection throughout the day, and before going to sleep. Review interactions, responses, events, lessons, and challenges from the day. Ask and answer the questions: 'What did I learn? 'What will I do differently?" "How did I contribute to the highest good?" Reflect. Resolve. Renew.

***Turn inward for strength, power, protection, peace, clarity, wisdom, and infinite Love.***

Develop, trust, and follow intuition – direct knowledge. Intuition is an inner knowing beyond conscious reasoning that is unlocked as we heal, evolve, and pay attention to all that is being communicated to us from both inner and outer worlds. Intuition can help us make a decision, choose a path, be forewarned, avoid danger, heal, reach our highest potential, and be happy. Intuitive Intelligence always supports evolution of the soul. Intuition always supports our highest good and will never lead us astray. Listening to and following Intuitive Intelligence is essential for optimizing health, happiness, and personal power, and for minimizing pain and suffering.

***Always trust innate wisdom.***

Intuitive information from all sources is received differently for every individual. Intuitive information from the brain is different from information from the heart and from the gut. Information can be in the form of thoughts, visions, premonitions, flashes of inspiration, feelings, sensations, warmth, music, sounds, symbols, and downloads. Intuitive power is increased by tuning into, trusting, and acting upon inner knowingness – by following gut instincts, inspirations, heart whispers, and/or paying attention to dreams and signs. When you trust what you receive, you are activating innate Dvinity. Trusting intuition strengthens intuition and facilitates healing, empowerment, sovereignty, and soul evolution.

*"It is then that you will hear a voice within yourself. It was there all along, but you never listened before. Faintly it will speak to you at first, but it will gradually grow louder and clearer the more you take heed of its' message, until one day it thunders inside you, and you will have come home."*
— Kristin Zambucka[42]

Develop empathy and compassion by caring, helping, sharing, listening to, and uplifting those in need. Share joy, positivity, encouragement, enthusiasm, optimism, and Love. Identify and reinforce positive qualities in others. Be generous with heartfelt compliments.

Deepen in relationship with All That Is. Fall in love with God, Divine Mother, Nature, Earth, planets, spirit guides, angels, Masters, crossed-over loved ones, animal and plant spirits, extraterrestrial/interdimensional family members, other/future selves, and other higher intelligences. Revel in intimate union with the Divine and explore the Divine romance. Use intuition,

---

[42] Zambucka, K. *Ano Ano; The Seed.* Mana Publishing, HI. 1978

imagination, persistence, patience, vigilance, discernment, common sense, and invoke protection from evil.

Establish and maintain heart-brain coherence – harmonious synchronization of the energies of the heart, mind, body, and Earth. There are simple techniques that one can use to create coherence, which can be practiced to establish heart-centeredness as a way of being.[43] Without heart-brain coherence, thoughts will tend to be scattered, clouded, negative, and extreme; physical activity will tend to be ineffective, destructive, or aggressive, even violent; bodily functions will be disrupted; and the energy of Life will dissipate. Living in coherence improves immune function, activates DNA, promotes longevity, facilitates downloads, and changes reality. It is highly beneficial to focus attention on feeling, creating, amplifying, and radiating love in the heart, and to strengthen that feeling at every opportunity.

***Begin the practice by relaxing, breathing slowly and deeply, and bringing to mind a loved one/pet/place/time. Focus your awareness on the feeling generated in your heart. Touching the heart center in the middle of the chest may help. One may feel warmth, softness, tenderness, tingling, spaciousness, Love, passion, and/or fire. Allow that feeling to expand and radiate out from the heart center with every breath. Continue for as long as desired.***

---

[43] www.hearthmath.org

Heart coherence is created, strengthened, and established by this practice and by being of service and performing kind and helpful actions, being creative, being peaceful, and being in Nature. We can use this ancient technique any time to reconnect with Infinite Intelligence, with Love, with peace, and with Truth. It can be used for decision-making, to relieve fear and anxiety, to rebalance, to increase personal power, and to return Home. We are most powerful when we live with heart coherence. Lead with your heart. Following your heart is empowering.[44] Turn your heart toward the light of God for optimal power and nourishment.

> *"Grandfather says: When you feel powerless, that's because you stopped listening to your own heart, that's where power comes from."*
> – Gianni Crow

Make Life sacred. Deepen in reverence for the gift of Life. Cultivate sacredness in all actions and activities. Bless everyone and everything, including oneself. Make your home/room a temple. Make and tend an altar or two. It is important to have a focus for one's devotion, prayers, Love, and spiritual practices. Personal power develops over time through devotion, prayers, offerings, and rituals. An offering is a gesture of appreciation, a demonstration of love, an act of devotion and humility, and a show of faith. Every heartfelt offering builds trust and faith in self and God and deepens our connection to All That Is. Making

---

[44] www.heartmath.org

offerings creates and amplifies energy that empowers our intentions and prayers. Making offerings raises our vibration, and the vibration of the surrounding space and beyond. In this sanctuary, one feels safe, protected, held, supported, loved, and guided. Offerings are part of the cycle of giving and receiving that sustains us. Heartfelt offerings can be made anywhere, at any time, in any way. Consider offering what feels meaningful: Flowers. Flower petals. Incense. Food. Fruits, Sprouting seeds. Water. Milk. Tobacco. Flames, Currency. Salt. Music. Songs. Ash. Tears. Blood. Self. Life.

> *"Wisdom is the sun of the soul, health is the sun of the body, and faith is the spiritual sun. The faith factor is the supreme energy factor of all.*
> *There is nothing in the Universe that strengthens as much as faith or allows strength to flow through it. There is nothing that weakens the human being or any social structure more than lack of faith. All fear arises, ultimately, from lack of faith."*
> – Manly P. Hall[45]

Develop faith and trust in a higher power/God/Love. Eliminate doubt. Trust that prayers will be answered, protection is provided, all needs will be met, and the way

---

[45] YouTube: *Organizing And Conserving Personal Energy Resources - Manly P. Hall, Full Lecture*, MindPodNetwork. 8 July 2019.
https://www.youtube.com/watch?v=A3aHeaODoJE

forward will be made clear. Trust that Love is the intelligent force of Creation, and all that unfolds is for the highest good of all. Trust the Divine Plan. Faith is the armor of God.

> *"The Divine Plan calls for a beautiful world – a world in which people are happy, useful, and able to achieve emotional fulfillment through the proper expression of affection, friendship, co-operation, and integrity."*
> – MANLY P. HALL[46]

Connect with benevolent ancestors. Our ancestors are wanting and waiting to communicate and to be of service. All their highest hopes, deepest heartfelt intentions, and noblest deeds have culminated in the life we are now living. Our ancestors are heavily invested in supporting us to evolve and to thrive as sovereign, Divine beings, because our evolutionary journeys are interlaced. Communicate/talk with ancestors and build relationships with all relations. Study family history. Respect the wisdom of elders. Appreciate earthly roots and galactic heritage. Make and tend an ancestor altar. Feel the power of the ancestors within. Draw upon their strength. Listen for their wisdom. Honor and respect ancestors by following their trail, dedicating oneself to living as an embodiment of Divine Love, and blazing a trail for others to follow.

---

[46] YouTube: *How To Find Your True Purpose, Manly P. Hall - Alchemy – Metaphysics – Philosophy*, MindPodNetwork, 2 October 2019. https://www.youtube.com/watch?v=EGhrhe1YAn4.

***You are the living hope of all your ancestors.***

Prayer is a superpower. Prayer increases personal power. There are countless benevolent beings waiting to connect, help, guide, teach, and participate in our evolution, which benefits their evolution. There are beings here now and civilizations throughout the Cosmos that are intrinsically connected to the evolution of the human race. Their evolution is dependent upon our evolution. With great humility, reverence, respect, and gratitude, one can ask for help from God, angels, ancestors, guides, and other higher intelligences, and help will be forthcoming. Beings of Love can only be of assistance when asked and will always provide assistance, often in ways that may never be known or understood. Pray for the Truth to be revealed, for health, for harmony, and for peace. Praying for protection from Evil provides protection from loss of personal power. The greatest protection from Evil is living life in service to God/good, being grounded and connected to Nature, practicing loving kindness, and undertaking actions to raise one's vibration, uplift our shared reality, expand Love, and serve Truth.

Practicing gratitude increases personal power. Feel grateful for everything that happens and does not happen. For blessings, Grace, beauty, peace, wellbeing, and miracles. And for challenges. Every moment is a gift, which is why the now moment is called the Present. Feeling grateful for challenging and painful life events further increases personal power and alleviates suffering over time. Express gratitude for sustenance, air, food, water, shelter, friends, possessions,

May all beings be
free from danger.

May all beings be
safe and protected.

May all beings be
free from suffering.

May all beings have
ease and well-being.

May all beings be free.

**Please and Thank You.**

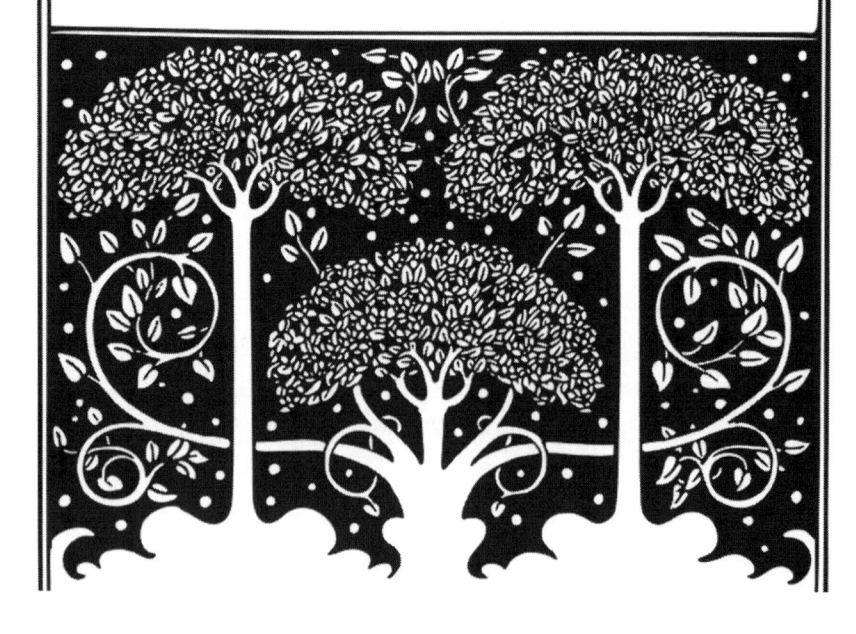

a beating heart, a free and clear mind, optimal health, healing, love and support from unseen beings, and for Life itself. Expressing gratitude for Nature while feeling the power of Nature promotes greater assimilation of Nature's bounty, beauty, and power. Develop an attitude of gratitude. Express gratitude frequently, both silently and aloud. Make mental lists and keep a gratitude journal.

Practice kindness. The keys to infinite Divine power and wisdom will never be accessed by anyone who is unkind, dishonest, selfish, and/or living out of integrity with Cosmic Spiritual Law. Intend to alleviate suffering and ignorance of self and others and take actions that do so. Identify when there is a need, an opportunity to alleviate human suffering and ignorance, and shine Light in the darkness. We are empowered by helping, serving, caring for, and uplifting others. Root yourself in kindness. Practicing random acts of kindness increases personal power.

***By empowering others, we empower ourselves.***

Develop patience. Practice being patient to develop patience and power. There are no shortcuts. Trust Divine timing.

Practice positive emotions: Joy. Gratefulness. Peacefulness. Contentment. Optimism. Enthusiasm. Positive emotions charge the mind and body with dynamic energy, which improves physical, mental, and social health, increases vitality and longevity, and strengthens personal power.

***Positivity builds personal power.***

Develop integrity. Integrity is the highest form of wealth and power. Your integrity is your superpower and your security. Align thoughts, words, and actions with Truth and with the principles of Natural Law. Speak truthfully, without manipulation, exaggeration, or deceit. Stop lying to other people and, most importantly, to yourself. Lying decreases personal power and destroys physical, mental, social, and spiritual health. Truthfulness is necessary for the acquisition of true, Divine power and higher knowledge. Apologize and make amends when necessary. Seek the restoration of wholeness whenever it has been lost. Say "yes" when you mean "yes," and "no" when you mean "no." Keep your word. Always be on time. Your time is no more important than another's. Develop humility or the Universe with do it for you! The spiritual ego is the wiliest of all. There will be endless initiations, lessons, and tests. Develop the willingness to rise above that which holds you back.

**A pure heart is forged in the fire of Life.**

Be vigilant for communications from God, Higher Self, Higher Intelligences, Nature, and from the physical body. Notice signs, symbols, synchronicities, co-incidences, and dreams. Those who learn to navigate through dreamscapes will have a greater advantage in life and upon death. Notice visions, downloads,[47] insights, conversations, song lyrics,

---

[47] A "download" is the receipt of information and higher knowledge from Infinite Intelligence.

music, animals, signs, and synchronicities. Notice bodily sensations, physical symptoms, impulses, inspirations, and inklings.

***Infinite Intelligence is always communicating. Are you listening?***

Be empowered by others. Find a mentor. Join a community or group of like-minded people with shared interests/goals for support, and to develop a sense of belonging with people who are kind, loving, honest, integrous, optimistic, generous, encouraging, and supportive.

Study Natural Law, Astrology, Alchemy, and other occult sciences. Read, listen to, and study ancient sacred texts.[48] Learn from ancient and indigenous wisdom traditions. Teaching higher knowledge increases personal power. Appreciate sacred art and artifacts, and indigenous art, medicines, and creation mythologies. Read ecstatic poetry. Study Astronomy, Symbology, Sacred Geometry, Permaculture, and Biodynamic Gardening. Learn from history. Appreciate Crop Circles, which are life-affirming codes that speak to the subconscious mind and DNA and repair our electromagnetic field (or aura).

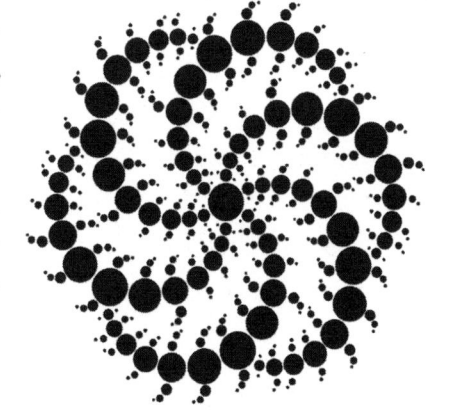

---

[48] https://www.sacred-texts.com/

Simplify Life. Simplicity is power. The more complicated the lifestyle, the more energy is expended and wasted. Simplicity conserves life-force energy. Minimize desires and live a life of moderation and contentment. Living in a clean, uncluttered, beautiful environment facilitates grace and power.

*Reduce. Reuse. Recycle. Repurpose. Repair. Donate. Repeat.*

Activating the alchemical/transformational power of cleaning increases personal power. By holding the intention to be cleansed, healed, uplifted, and relieved of all that no longer serves one's highest good, inner transformation takes place while cleaning. Cleaning on the outside cleans on the inside. As above, so below. Clean, beautify, and cherish: Body. Mind. Home. Clothes. Car. Workspace. Public places. Wild places. Cleanliness is Godliness.

**Walk in beauty and create beauty wherever you go.**

Invoke your "genius" – the genie-in-us. Everybody is a genius. Appreciate the genius of Infinite Intelligence at every opportunity. Practice magic. Everybody is a magician and an alchemist. Magic is the ability to create changes in consciousness at will. Magic can be used for self-transformation and to increase the likelihood of a desired future outcome coming into physical reality. Practicing magic should only be done for the highest good of all. This is white magic, No good comes from using magic and harnessing cosmic power to serve self. Any selfish use of magic for personal gain is black magic, which brings more pain, suffering, and evil into this world.

Combine the power of mind, heart, will, and Infinite Intelligence with sounds, symbols, allies, and actions to create, manifest, and transform in powerful ways. Magic supports action, and action supports magic. Create a circle of power and protection. Create ceremonies and rituals to empower prayers, intentions, and actions that contribute the highest good of all. Create a morning ritual to begin each day in gratitude and in service to God. Create talismans and amulets for protection and to increase personal power and collective power. Silence helps to keep something sacred.

> ***The magic works through you.***
> ***Not beside you. Not around you,***
> ***but through you.***
> ***Let your life be your wand."***
> – UNKNOWN

It is empowering to imagine oneself as a beacon of blindingly brilliant Light/Love, radiating out and engulfing All That Is in a tsunami of opalescent Lifeforce energy that extends out from and back into the heart center in a double torus of energy. Projecting our natural energy field in this way and moving beyond fear and all emotions of a lower nature are extremely powerful ways to change reality. Radiating and pulsating rainbow light is another powerful practice to change reality. (See following diagram).

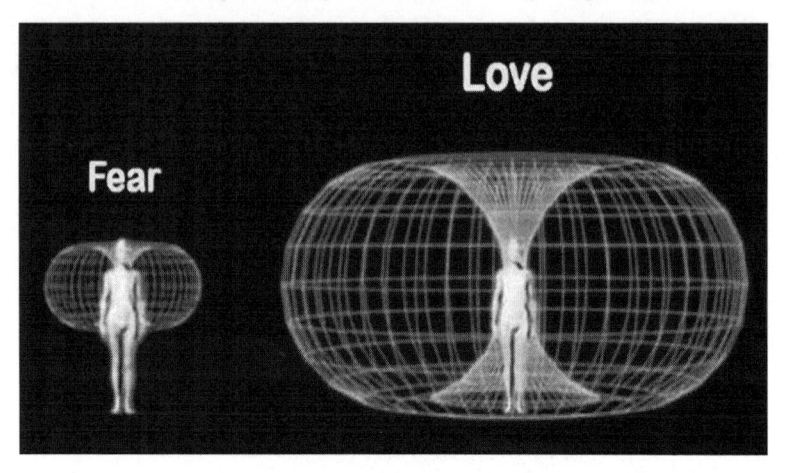

**Fear**

**Love**

Learn about and activate your Light Body, which is a sacred, geometric hologram of Divine Love; an ascension vehicle; a chariot of light for the soul; and a source of power and protection. A light body is also known as a Merkabah – 'Mer' (Light), 'Ka' (Spirit), 'Bah' (Body). Information about the existence and purpose of the Merkabah has been intentionally occulted to keep humans powerless, enslaved, and trapped in the endless cycle of reincarnation here on Earth. Each of us has a Merkabah, a crystalline energy field, that extends approximately 17 meters (55 feet)) from the body when it is fully activated. It is comprised of specific sacred geometries that align the mind, body, and heart with Love.

The light body can be envisioned as a star tetrahedron - two interlocked tetrahedrons, a three-dimensional Star of David - that are counter-rotating fields of light and energy surrounding every human being.[49] These geometric energy fields normally spin around our bodies at close to the speed of light, but for most of us, they have slowed down considerably – or stopped spinning entirely – due to a lack of awareness and fear, which destroys the Light body. When this field is reactivated, reenergized, and spinning properly, it is known as a Merkabah. (See diagram.)

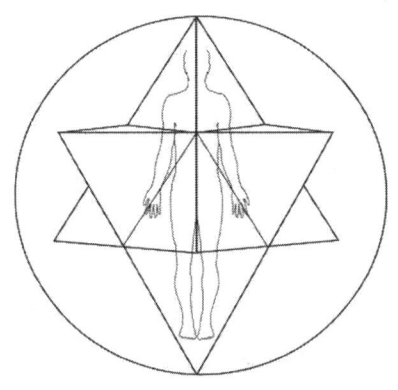

The light body can be a source of creative power and enlightenment. The Merkabah fluidly integrates our feminine (intuitive, receptive) aspects and masculine (active, dynamic) aspects and brings us into wholeness. Within the Merkabah, spiritual and psychic power is greatly increased. The Merkabah enables us to experience expanded awareness, connect with elevated potentials of consciousness, and restore memory of and access to the infinite possibilities of our being. It can help one to realize one's full potential and connect with innate Divinity, goodness, compassion, empathy, Truth, and Divine Love. This field of Light, Love, harmony, and goodwill extends to others and envelops them in Love and healing energy. In this way, we co-author each other's biology and uplift Humanity.

---

[49] It is important to note that the Merkabah is an individual expression of energy that can be any shape and size.

# LOVE is POWER

*Unconditional Love has infinite power to heal. Be the ripple.*

The Merkabah can be used take us beyond this physical embodiment, transcend this Earthly reality, and travel to other dimensions and realities while we are physically embodied. A Merkabah can be activated and strengthened with intention and attention, using meditation, visualizations, breathwork, spinning, dancing, fasting, frequencies, and other sacred practices. The Merkabah can be recreated and activated with intuition, Love, Faith, and Will.

A Merkabah will protect from evil. Establishing protection from Evil is also achieved using will, intentions, prayer, a declaration of sovereignty, and visualizations. One can imagine oneself inside a Merkabah, a ball of brilliant light, or a sphere that has a mirrored outer surface. Hold the intention that whatever is being directed to you that is not for your highest good be redirected toward higher levels of consciousness and Love.

Create a balance between inner/spiritual life, domestic life, private life, and public life. Balance is the key to true power.

Prepare for death. How you die is as important as how you live. Leave this world a better person and leave this world a better place. There is no hell other than self-imposed hell. Hell is an invention of religions to instill fear and control humans.

Create a vision for the future – for humankind, for self, for New Earth. How does it feel? How does it look? This is how we co-create a safe, peaceful, abundant, and beautiful place for Humanity to thrive. Stay focused on a clear seed picture and energize this vision as a priority. In every sense, feel that New Earth is already here because it is. Until the seed bears fruit, hold it close so as not to spill its power to reach fruition. Erase doubt, which will cause the seed picture to wither and die.

> "Heal yourself with the light of the Sun and the rays of the Moon. With the sound of the river and the waterfall. With the swaying of the sea and the fluttering of birds. Heal yourself with mint, neem, and eucalyptus. Sweeten with lavender, rosemary, and chamomile. Hug yourself with the cocoa bean and a hint of cinnamon. Put love in tea instead of sugar and drink it looking at the stars. Heal yourself with the kisses that the wind gives you and the hugs of the rain. Stand strong with your bare feet on the ground and with everything that comes from it. Be smarter every day by listening to your intuition, looking at the world with your forehead and heart. Jump, dance, sing, so that you live happier. Heal yourself, with beautiful love, and always remember ...
>
> You are the Medicine."
>
> \- Maria Sabina

# WHAT TO AVOID

Avoid abusing and misusing personal power. Avoid doing harm to other sentient beings. No killing, lying, stealing, hurting, raping, controlling, manipulating, abusing, bullying, bullshitting, mindfuckery, coercion, or violating free will. No wasting the energy or attention of another person. No animal cruelty, inhumane slaughter of animals, sport hunting, trophy hunting, sport fishing, or animal experimentation.

Avoid and eliminate mind viruses. Weitkio[50] is a highly contagious, highly deceptive, self-replicating mind-virus that has infected Humanity through our collective unconsciousness and threatens the survival of humankind. Weitko is a psycho-spiritual disease of the soul that drives insatiable consumption, narcissism, and the pandemic of selfishness that threatens our future. Wetiko is a collective psychosis that operates through self-deception and effects our ability to think, see, and act in ways that support our own good and the common good. Wetiko acts through a blind spot in the psyche and generates negative hallucinations and reactions that do not serve the highest good and compels human beings to act in ways that are self-destructive, inhumane, and insane. Weitko feeds off fear, anxiety, anger, hatred, sadness, guilt, shame, confusion, conflict, polarization, pain, lies, and suffering. Weitiko is perpetuated

---

[50] Weitko (Alogonquin noun): a cannibalistic spirit that is driven by greed, excess, and selfish consumption. It deludes its host into believing that cannibalizing the life-force energy of others (including animals and other lifeforms) is a logical and morally upright way to live.
Levy, P. *Dispelling Wetiko: Breaking the Curse of Evil*. North Atlantic Books. USA. 2018. https://www.awakeninthedream.com/

by selfishness, ignorance, arrogance, and cowardice.

Cognitive dissonance is a symptom of Weitiko. Most people on Earth are suffering from cognitive dissonance now that the evil of once-trusted social systems is being exposed. Cognitive dissonance is the state of having inconsistent, contradictory, conflicting, and nonsensical thoughts, beliefs, and/or attitudes about self, life, and the nature of reality. People who hold fast to unexamined beliefs are suffering from cognitive dissonance. We are in the experience of a collective psychosis of evil of epic proportions, and this is the real pandemic.

Avoid feeling like a victim. At our soul's request, Life happens for us, not to us. Avoid blaming others, making excuses, and ascribing life events to luck, chance, and karma. Take full responsibility for all that unfolds in Life – personally and collectively. For all creations, all actions and reactions, and all inactions and omissions. For all thoughts, feelings, and needs. For all choices and their consequences. It is very disempowering to blame others and/or expect them to meet personal needs. Verbalizing blame reinforces victimhood. Until one takes full responsibility for oneself and all of one's creations, Divine power remains a concept, rather than an activated principle. Self-responsibility *is* self-empowerment.

Avoid fear, anxiety, and confusion, which destroy mental and physical health. Avoid TV, news, fear porn, misery porn, and doom scrolling. Avoid fear of death. There is no death. Life is eternal. We are immortal, energetic beings of Light. Energy cannot be destroyed. It can only change form. Death is a transition from a physical to a non-physical state. Instilling fear of death in humans is arguably the most disempowering tactic used to oppress and enslave humankind. This lie keeps humans living in fear, and fearful humans are controllable and ideal sustenance for parasitic lifeforms.

***Do not become their food.***
***Do not feed the beast system.***

Another lie that has been inserted into the collective consciousness to ensure continuous and copious sustenance for the parasites is the notion that ending one's life is wrong and leads to eternal hell and damnation. As the master of one's own soul and destiny, the choice to end one's earthly life is entirely between oneself and Infinite Intelligence, and has nothing to do with doctors, priests, family members, man's laws, and man's traditions. There is no one judging or punishing you other than yourself. All fear and taboo around suicide is generated and perpetuated to keep people here on Earth, living in fear, suffering for years, sometimes decades, afraid to free themselves and go Home.

The life we are living is ours to do with as we choose. Live or die? It is your life and your creation, and the choice to end one's earthly life is always and only a personal choice. You chose when where, how, and why you came into this incarnation, and you can choose when, where, how, and why you exit. It is your life and your death, and you are answerable to no-one other than yourself. The choice to end one's life is one that can be made at any time without negative consequences for the soul, because every experience is an opportunity for learning and evolution. The decision to stop suffering, stop contributing negative energy to the collective consciousness, and stop feeding dark forces – who are the only beneficiaries from human suffering – is yours, and yours, alone. There is no reason to wait for a "natural death" if one is suffering. All opposition to the individual choice to die is evil. Prolonging the lives of those who are suffering and have no quality of life is both evil and profitable.

Avoid worrying. Do not worry about things over which you have no control. Worry is destructive emotion and wasted energy. Worry undermines faith and power. Choose to strengthen faith in God/self/Love.

Avoid all Spiritual teachers, New Age/ New Thought leaders, and religious leaders who do not teach Natural Law/Cosmic Spiritual Law. Avoid those with an audience or platform who do not bring attention to the enslavement of Humanity and the hijacking of our organic reality and our natural timeline. There is a jackboot standing on the neck of humankind, and far too many "influencers" are using their platform for self-promotion, self-gratification, and mental masturbation, rather than addressing the most pressing issues of our time. Seek information from those who teach Natural Law and provide clear information on how to free oneself, how to thrive as a sovereign being, how to serve God, and how to co-create and live on New Earth – the Love-based reality of beauty and bounty that is our birthright.

***Anyone with a platform who is not raising the alarm about the tyranny of Evil enslaving Humanity, or calling for a peaceful uprising,***

*and/or sharing information about
how to thrive as a sovereign being,
is either brainwashed, braindead,
or complicit, and a servant of Evil.
Anyone who is preaching about Truth, Freedom,
and Unity who has taken or recommends
the death jab is a fraud, a sellout,
and servant of Evil.*

Avoid those who claim to have a special connection to God, to be an intermediary, a representative, or a mouthpiece for God. Avoid those who claim they know what God wants/thinks/plans and what is best for you. Avoid those who claim to have "inside information" or higher knowledge from a "source that cannot be named."

Avoid any information, teachings, and teachers that speak of a savior or a team of saviors. No one and nothing is coming to save us. The lie about a Savior coming to our rescue is one of the most disempowering lies that has been implanted into the collective consciousness. Savior programming makes people passive, cowardly, and firmly attached to the false reality matrix of enslavement.

*"There is no savior save self."*
— MAGENTA PIXIE[51]

---

[51] www.magentapixie.com

Freedom comes only through intention, effort, and actions. Freedom is an inside job. One must be prepared to take full responsibility for oneself, do the spiritual/inner work, heal emotional wounds[52], and illuminate all shadows.[53] One must be willing to go through the dark night of the soul. In order to be free and empowered, one must take full responsibility for all thoughts, words, actions, and creations, and for making changes to ensure that all thoughts, words, actions, and creations are in alignment with Natural Law and contribute to the alleviation of suffering and the upliftment and liberation of humankind.

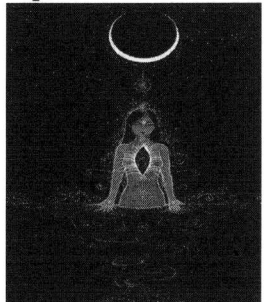

*"Only those who have the courage to walk in darkness can be as bright as the Sun and the Moon."*

– Eva Wong[54]

---

[52] Emotional wounds are inflicted from abuse, abandonment, betrayal, fear, loss, and trauma in childhood. Unhealed wounds are known as emotional baggage because they drain personal power. 90% of our energy is being used to suppress emotional baggage. Inner work/emotional healing is necessary to optimize personal power and end multigenerational trauma..

[53] Parts of oneself that are hidden, denied, suppressed, considered ugly, unacceptable, unconscious, subconscious, and running the show – fear, anger, guilt, shame, selfishness, greed, envy, childhood wounds, traumas, insecurities, embarrassments, neuroses, compulsions, fetishes, addictions, inauthenticities, and secrets. Facing fears, doing shadow work, wrestling inner demons, and healing emotional wounds from abuse and trauma brings freedom and power and never stops.

[54] YouTube: *Being Taoist: Wisdom for Living a Balanced Life by Eva Wong.* [FULL AUDIOBOOK REMASTERED AUDIO]. Spiritual Audiobooks, 9 March 2021. https://www.youtube.com/watch?v=eOmuIBEEyMk

Avoid those who teach others how to use personal power to "get what you want" and "create the life you want." This is selfish/evil misuse of personal power. The highest use of personal power is to live Life in service to God, and to use personal power, as directed by God, to serve the greater good, the highest good, the common good. Pay attention to those who teach that the best use of personal power is to serve God and Truth and to uplift Humanity. Through serving God/good, one's heart's desires are fulfilled, and infinite power is activated.

Avoid all those who stand between oneself and God. No-one needs an intermediary, a priest, a rabbi, or a guru. Beware of those claiming to be a "master" or "enlightened." Beware the hordes of dangerous deceivers along the spiritual path offering redemption, salvation, forgiveness, interpretations, predictions, deceptions, half-truths, and endless diversions and distractions to those seeking God, Truth, and self-mastery. Use discernment, because kind-hearted, well-intentioned human beings are the easiest to manipulate and take advantage of. Many who present themselves as spiritual teachers, religious leaders, gurus, evolved souls, New Thought Leaders, Ascension Guides, healers, Light Workers, channelers, and insiders privy to higher knowledge are servants of themselves – masterful manipulators, deceitful distractors, and instruments of Evil. We can look forward to escalating exposures of these sycophants.

Avoid distractions from being here now. Cultivate moment-to-moment awareness. Practice mindfulness. Slow down. Attend to one thing at a time. Notice breathing and bodily sensations. Notice thoughts and feelings. Observe inner and outer states. The ability to exist in the present moment in an aware, non-judgmental, patient, and sustained way has been shown to have many health benefits. Mindful individuals tend to have reduced stress levels, improved focus, inner and relational harmony, and they are less emotionally reactive.

While information about the past, present, and future and other timelines and realities is endlessly fascinating, it is important to stay present and fully embodied to effect the greatest change. Avoid mindless entertainment, endless screen time, reality analyses, and virtual rabbit holes of information that have been created to waste our time and attention and decrease power, health, joy, creativity, and vitality. Avoid all weapons of mass distraction, most notably the screens, the evil clown shows, and fabricated dramas playing out on the world stage. Avoid being ungrounded, out of body, and off-planet.

Avoid squandering sexual energy. There is no greater power than the power of sexual energy, also known as Kundalini. Increasing personal power through harnessing sexual energy is the most occulted and dangerous knowledge because this power creates everything and anything. Arousal is a superpower. Human beings are directed and encouraged to squander, misuse, and pervert sexual energy into extremely low vibrational energy that feeds the parasites: Pornography.[55]

---

[55] Pornography is a weapon, which causes brain damage. Viewing porn damages dopamine receptors, which leads to low testosterone, anxiety, depression, decreased self-confidence, reduced motivation, and addiction. Porn disconnects the viewer from reality and destroys the relationship between

Promiscuity. Misogyny. Deviancy. Sexual violence. Pedophilia. Sexualization of children. Gender dysphoria.

Avoid excessive sexual activity, desires, and fantasies, which deplete Lifeforce energy. Those who let their sexual desires run wild are destroying their bodies. Fantasized sexual activity can deplete generative energy as much as physical sex. Having sex when you are angry, sad, fearful, and drunk disrupts the harmony of Humanity. Forced celibacy can lead to abnormal and harmful sexual behaviors, mental instability, and a reduced lifespan. The key to a healthy sex life lies in regulation, moderation, and self-discipline. Making sexuality sacred and making Love increases personal power and decreases the power of Evil on Earth. Self-pleasuring and making love with the intention of offering orgasmic energy to serve the common good is an empowering practice. There are many powerful practices from Ancient Wisdom/Tantric traditions that teach responsible use of sexual energy to improve personal health, personal power, and the well-being of all.

> **Before lovemaking and self-pleasuring,
> make a silent or spoken offering:
> "Please amplify this Love.
> May it bless and uplift all life on Earth
> and throughout the Cosmos."**

Offering Love energy in this way in this way is a superpower. Avoid lust, promiscuity, and perversions. Avoid men and women making it easier to control the population.

participating in violent sex, including BDSM,[56] which is an egregious misuse of Divine power. Creating pain and suffering is evil, with consent or lack thereof. Avoid playing violent games and violent video games. Avoid watching horror movies, violent movies, end-of-world movies, the news, and pornography. The subconscious mind cannot tell the difference between a "real"/actual experience and a virtual experience. All these genres generate low vibrational energy, which keeps an individual in fear, unbalanced, confused, angry, suffering, and feeding forces of evil. The same is true for low-vibrational music, literature, and all sources of information that increase fear and confusion, diminish personal power, prevent expansion of consciousness, and manifest a dark reality.

Avoid tattoos and body piercings that can serve as portals for negative entities. Choose wisely and invoke protection.

Avoid living with clutter, mess, filth, and being physically unclean. Live more fully and freely with fewer things that evoke more joy.

Avoid hatred, revenge, spite, slander, mockery, bitterness, envy, possessiveness, jealousy, arrogance, competitiveness, pride, greed, and desire, which are poisonous emotions that deplete the mind of dynamic energy; decrease physical, mental, and social health; destroy happiness, vitality, and longevity; and weaken personal power. These emotions create sickness, weakness, aggression, anxiety, and suffering, and render one unable to respond to life events with clarity, reason,

---

[56] BDSM – Bondage/Discipline, Dominance/Submission, Sadism/Masochism.

and strength. Withholding joy in the heart for blessings received by others withholds blessings from oneself. It is very empowering to acknowledge the achievements of others and celebrate when other people experience good/positive/uplifting life events.

***Love fearlessly, fiercely, unapologetically, and unconditionally,***
***like your life depends on it.***
***Because it does.***

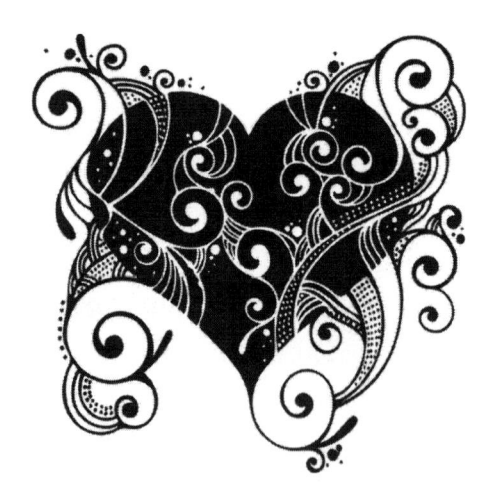

# INCREASING MENTAL POWER

*"All things, all of life, all of creation,
is part of One Original Thought.
You are part of the Original Thought." - Ra*

***You are creating the future with your
thoughts, words, and actions.
How you think, speak, and act today
becomes the fabric of reality tomorrow.***

Consciousness is energy. All that exists has arisen from consciousness. Every manifested thing is a trinity of consciousness, energy, and matter. A thought contains energy, substance, intelligence, and direction. Matter coalesces around frequency. Thoughts coagulate matter. Our thoughts create our reality. Our thoughts, beliefs, and imaginations are the creative force of our collective reality. Intention and attention create manifestations in physical and non-physical realities. Thinking is creating. Dark thoughts create dark reality. New Earth is being created by thoughts of Love, peace, joy, harmony, beauty, anarchy, and equality. Be vigilant.

Our thoughts make us who we are – conscious thoughts and those buried in the subconscious mind. The subconscious mind stores experiences from birth and delivers programmed and patterned responses accordingly. The subconscious mind is a garden and knows only to create reality from the seeds of thought. Sow good, moral, loving, uplifting, beautiful, and selfless thoughts, and reap benefits. Sow negative, selfish, immoral, and evil thoughts, and suffer. Know the truth about who you are and your inherent Divinity. You are an immortal, spiritual being having a very temporary, temporal experience. You are Divine in nature with infinte power and potential. You are a soverign soul - sacrosanct and ungovernable. If you believe you are separate from God, you will be as weak and alone as if you truly are.

**You are what you think you are.**
**Believe you will be well, and you will be.**
**Believe you are sick, and you will be.**
**Believe you are all-powerful, and you are.**
**Believe you are free, and you are.**
**It is done. So be it.**

Be the keen observer of your own thought processes. Notice thoughts as they arise and stop/derail all negative/fearful/false "thought trains" within 17 seconds before they gather momentum to avoid negative consequences. Deny all fear-based, critical, destructive, self-deprecating, non-loving thoughts, which are lies and illusions and have no existence in Truth. Replace negative thoughts with positive, neutral, constructive, uplifting, peaceful, empowering, truthful, loving thoughts. Change how you think to change your life.

**Policing thoughts is a full-time job.**

Optimizing brain health is essential. Detoxify the brain, Decalcify and open the pineal gland (the Third Eye). Eliminate fluoride and all neurotoxins. Protect the brain from physical, electromagnetic, and frequency damage. Balance brain hemispheres. Stay grounded. Sungaze. Practice relaxation. Optimize sleep. Exercise daily. Improve dental health to improve mental health. Optimize brain fuel. The optimal brain fuel is healthy fats.[57]

Learn how to learn, how to think clearly and critically, and how to reason. Study the Trivium and the Quadrivium[58] to get a unified idea of realty. Learn to think differently. Break through internal barriers, false dogmas, and self-imposed limitations. Go beyond your comfort zone and past known boundaries to find solutions and answers.

> ***"No problem can be solved by the same level of consciousness that created it."***
> – Albert Einstein

Develop the power of imagination. Imagination is everything. Imagination is an energy-producing, miracle force that activates the miracle response center in the brain – the Divine/Superconscious Mind. Through imagination, all things are created, and all things are possible. Imagination can be activated by meditating, daydreaming, being in Nature, being

---

[57] Sources of healthy fats include olive oil, avocado and avocado oil, hemp seeds and hemp seed oil, flaxseeds and flax seed oil, pumpkin seeds, sunflower seeds, chia seeds, coconut and coconut oil, MCT oil, organic butter, and nuts. Ensure all products are organic and sustainably sourced and harvested.

[58] YouTube: *Mark Passio – The Trivium*. The Mystic Trance, 2016. https://www.youtube.com/watch?v=SJ_X1SjmA5A&feature=youtu.be

curious, being playful, creating art, reading a book, doing new things, going to new places, participating in outdoor adventure activities, gardening, dream analysis and learning new skills.

Cultivate self-love and positive beliefs about self and about Life, particularly all that seems unlovable. Mirrorwork is a powerful way to establish and enhance self-love and undertake shadow work.[59] Develop an attitude of positive expectancy. Strive to establish a bright, cheerful, and optimistic attitude. Awaken creativity, playfulness, and childlike energy/childness. Be surrounded by objects, clothes, people, and colors that evoke love, peace, and joy. Practice self-care.

*Love yourself like your life depends on it,*
*because it does.*
*Love is the answer.*
*Love Light. Love Truth. Love Life.*

Be authentic. Be vulnerable. Vulnerability is strength. Be willing to take leaps into the unknown, learn from experiences, change course, and surrender to Divine Will. Seek soul growth,

---

[59] Mirrorwork is a powerful practice to develop self-love, self-respect, and self-forgiveness. By looking into a mirror and repeating "I love you," self-love can be established and deepened. Mirrorwork is based on the principle that our experience of life is mirrored by our relationship with our self. Cultivating a brutally honest, loving relationship with oneself cultivates deeply enriching life experiences. By looking into a mirror and softly focusing a loving, compassionate gaze into your eyes and repeating "I love myself" (or any other positive affirmation), self-love and self-confidence will arise, and an all-powerful connection with Source will be forged. Hay, Louise. *Mirrorwork: 21 Days to Heal Your Life*, Hay House Inc., USA. 2016.

emotional healing, expansion of consciousness, refinement, and wisdom. Strengthen mental stamina, resilience, tenacity, persistence, and will power. Life is challenging, and without mental strength, it is far more difficult to navigate steadily and confidently, to make tough decisions, and to weather the storms, the setbacks, the losses, the grief, the failures, and learn the lessons. Perseverance builds magnetic and electrical currents in the brain and body which charge the nerves and muscles with a super-abundance of dynamic energy that sources us through challenging times.

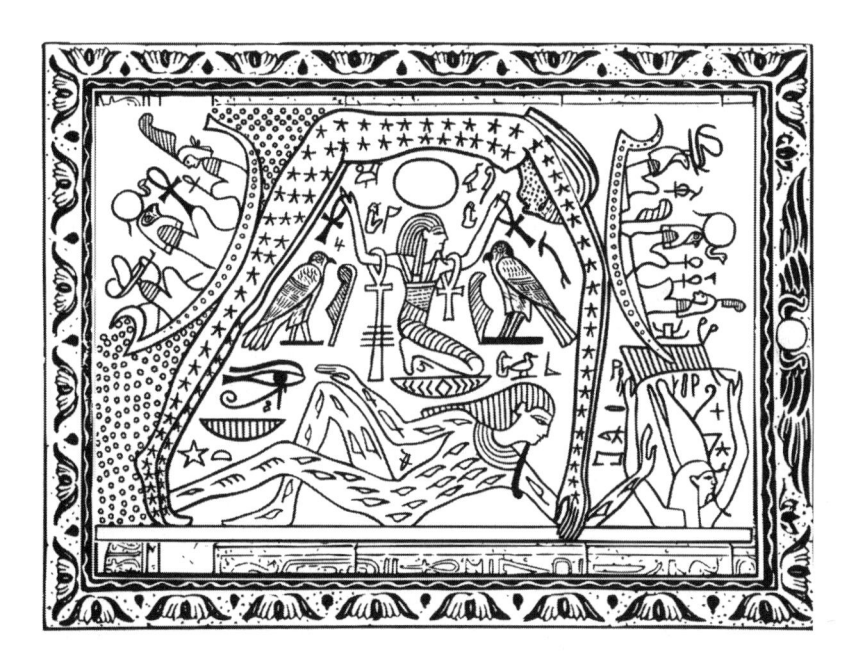

# ACTIONS TO STRENGTHEN WILL POWER

Will power is considered to have three components – the ability to do what is disagreeable; willing not to do something; and knowing what you want in the first place. The choice to focus the mind is the first step in harnessing mind power and increasing will power.

Meditation is an essential practice for focusing the power of the mind. Meditation turns awareness inward toward the intangible life of consciousness – the internal universe. Meditation is access to the infinite wealth of consciousness. Meditation dissolves duality and frees one from limitation. Meditation helps to cultivate a peaceful and powerful disposition.

Hold the intention to align Free Will with Divine Will.

**Let Thy Will be done through and unto me.**
**Please make me an instrument of Divine Will.**

Align thoughts, feelings, words, and actions with Love, live in integrity, and in harmony with Nature.

Listen to and act upon intuition. Pay attention to all communications from internal and external worlds.

Choose words wisely. Too many people squander personal power by squandering the power of speech. Excessive talking and arguing disrupts mental and physical health. Speak only when necessary and refrain from useless banter and needing to be right, which depletes personal power. Speaking words that are not fully understood and speaking without awareness is disempowering. We can speak words and make sounds that shape and structure matter and give us power (positive and uplifting words, tones, songs, chants, mantras, spells, and incantations). We can speak words and make sounds that weaken us (negative and fearful words, curse words, gossip, slander, complaining, scaremongering). Words change reality. For example, replacing "I can't" and "It's impossible" with "I can" and "Anything is possible" is empowering. Replacing "I have to" with "I get to" changes obligations into opportunities. Speak with confidence. Use positive language. Use Nonviolent Communication[60] and the Five Love Languages.[61] Study etymology and phonics.[62] Avoid polluting our shared reality and perpetuating the matrix of enslavement with irrelevancies, falsities, diatribes, and doom and gloom. Hold close secrets, visions, heartfelt intentions, and desires to contain power for fruition. Mystery has power.

Use positive self-talk and affirmations. "I am" is the most powerful statement one can make. What follows these two most powerful words is commanded into being and shapes our reality, so choose these words wisely. For example, it is infinitely more empowering to say "I feel sick," rather than "I am sick." Never own a disease. "I feel anger/sadness/hurt, and/or fearful," is empowering. "I am angry/sad/hurt, and/or fearful," is disempowering. Repeat positive statements like "I am safe,

---

[60] https://www.cnvc.org/

[61] https://www.5lovelanguages.com/

[62] https://www.etymonline.com/

free, courageous, healthy, powerful, and invincible. All is well." Act and feel free, courageous, healthy, and powerful in order to embody new, beneficial, and empowering ways of being.

Find a purpose or a passion that lights your inner fire. Igniting and fueling one's inner fire is key to increasing personal power. Find your own singularity. This is your responsibility. Set goals that are aligned with your purpose – daily and long-term. Do at least one thing to improve physical and mental health every day. Do at least one thing that contributes to spiritual growth every day. Do at least one thing that helps another person every day. Do at least one thing that contributes to the greater good every day. Be meticulous to ensure actions are aligned with purpose, which increases personal power.

Be disciplined. Stop wasting time and energy, procrastinating, or making excuses. If one does not practice self-discipline, suffering is ensured. Now is the time to be disciplined and focused with a definite purpose. There is no time to waste. Create a daily routine and stick to it. Direct focus and energy toward the betterment of all. Perform activities that serve God/ the highest good, that alleviate suffering and ignorance, and that are empowering, uplifting, good, moral, and in alignment with Natural Law. For example: performing random acts of kindness and anonymous charity; volunteering, helping people; feeding people, growing food, sharing food; caring for children, elders, plants, gardens, pets, and animals; cleaning, decluttering, picking up trash; planting trees and fruit trees, being creative, and creating beauty.

*"Hunger is the first element of self-discipline. If you can control what you eat and drink, you can control everything else."*
— Dr. Umar Faruq Abd-Allah

Doing what serves the highest good but may not be much fun at the time increases will power, such as washing dishes, making the bed, cleaning the toilet, and exercising when it is cold. Will power is strengthened when a challenging situation arises, and it is met without shirking and shrinking, but by reaching deep inside oneself, into one's essence, and doing what needs to be done. Will power is consolidated every time the choice is made to persevere and move through and beyond hardships, fear, and pain. Will power is forged every time one refuses to give up on self and Life. Will power is strengthened by setting an intention/goal of any size and achieving that intention/goal despite setbacks, problems, obstacles, and challenges. After being hurt, betrayed, abandoned, broken, and burned repeatedly, making the decision to rise up from the ashes requires enormous will power. Will power is strengthened by acting intuitively and courageously.

*"Nature loves courage. You make the commitment and Nature will respond to that commitment by removing impossible obstacles. Dream the impossible dream and the world will not grind you under, it will lift you up. This is the trick. This is what all these teachers and philosophers who really counted, who really*

> *touched the alchemical gold, this is what they understood. This is the shamanic dance in the waterfall. This is how magic is done. By hurling yourself into the abyss and discovering it's a feather bed."*
>
> – TERENCE MCKENNA

Question everything: Information. Identity. Motives. Purpose. Intent. Very few people question their life path, their purpose, or their ability to make choices about how to live fully and freely. We are limitless unless we limit ourselves. Examine mind programming and beliefs about self and Life to determine what is true and empowering and what is false, limiting, and disempowering. Changing beliefs that are disempowering to truths that are empowering is most effectively done through the subconscious mind. Hypnosis, autosuggestion, visualizations, repetition of new thought habits and behaviors, subliminal messages, affirmations, mantras, clinical hypnotherapy, biofeedback, Energy Psychology and Belief Changing Modifications, including EFT (tapping),[63] PSYCH-K, and EMDR (Eye Movement Desensitization and Reprocessing) can rewrite limiting and negative beliefs with new and empowering programming. Tapping (EFT) is an easy and powerful way to clear energy blocks, heal wounds, restore balance, and increase personal power, health, and well-being.

The subconscious mind is the default operating system

---

[63] www.thetappingsolution.com

when the conscious mind is thinking, which is approximately 95% of the time.[64] From very early in life, the subconscious mind records and stores memories, emotions, and experiences (everything we see, hear, think, and feel emotionally), which become fundamental operating programs from around seven years of age. The subconscious mind takes everything literally and does not distinguish between what is experienced and what is imagined. Our beliefs, values, habits, and behaviors are formed and directed by these subconscious programs, not all of which are beneficial or helpful. Any programs, thought patterns, and beliefs that limit our health, our abilities, our potential, our freedom, and our happiness need to be identified and reprogrammed with truths that promote optimal health and well-being, personal power, and sovereignty. Tapping into the power of the subconscious mind will unlock innate gifts, higher knowledge, and hidden potentials. The subconscious mind can be directed to access genius, solve problems, and guide life.

Keep learning. Will power is fortified by knowledge of Natural Law, Astrology, Earth energy, frequency, and self. There is always more to learn about self, consciousness, Truth, energy, and the nature of reality. It is naïve and dangerous to assume that one knows what is really going on. Be curious. Keep enlarging worldview, expanding consciousness, and broadening perception. Train the mind to perceive through sensory and extrasensory perceptions. Keep researching and reading books with paper pages. Keep a journal. Keep a dream

---

[64] YouTube: *Bruce Lipton: The Biology of Belief Full Lecture*. Vekmehel Ofkir, 2015. https://www.Youtube.com/watch?v=82ShSNuru6c.

journal. Write letters. Take the opportunity to learn a skill that brings joy, takes you out of your comfort zone, and/or helps you to help others. Be creative without an electronic device. Learn a handicraft, a language, a musical instrument, a poem, a song.

Keep raising your vibrational frequency. Our vibration is the secret of our inherent power.[65] The higher our vibration, the greater our power. Change your frequency to change your life experience. Continually release all that keeps one's vibration low and all that no longer serves the highest good – thoughts, beliefs, emotions, habits, addictions, behaviors, relationships, foods, drinks, drugs, possessions, social settings, jobs, environments, and teachers. Every time we clear and liberate ourselves in this way, Divine Essence floods our being and continues to raise our vibrational frequency ad infinitum Increasing one's vibration accelerates the destruction of the false reality matrix  Relax, breathe, be in Nature, sungaze, and stay grounded.

> *"Gnosis is self-emptying. We have to self-empty ourselves of all the blocks to make room for Christ energy."*
>
> – GEOFF THOMPSON[66]

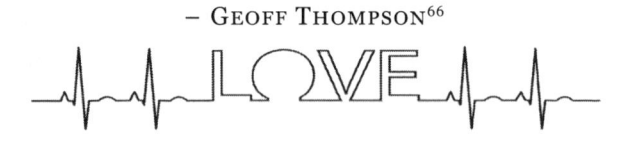

---

[65] YouTube: *20 Easy Ways to Raise Your Vibration: Essential Information for All Human Beings.* Feeling Better Naturally.18 December 2020. https://www.youtube.com/watch?v=H9yKlvevu1c

[66] YouTube: *Proper Selfishness, Overcoming Fear and Inner Work. In Conversation with Geoff Thompson.* Pat Divilly. 7 November 2020 https://www.youtube.com/watch?v=W7NsZWybsKY

Practice forgiveness. Forgiving is releasing a frequency of hatred that only affects oneself. Forgiveness happens through self-resolution – the decision to free oneself from destructive energetic connections to others, learn from experience, and return to center. Forgiveness happens toward oneself, not toward someone else. Forgiving another person for real or perceived wrongs is an empowering practice that does not need to be communicated or acted upon. Ultimately there is no-one to forgive other than oneself, because there are no victims. Those who hurt, betray, abandon, and abuse us are fulfilling the roles we agreed they would play in this lifetime to move us forward on our evolutionary journey. Everything that happens and does not happen is what we have chosen and created for our spiritual growth. Take ownership. Practice self-forgiveness and self-compassion. Forgiveness does not mean forgetting.

> *"I am sorry. Please forgive me.*
> *Thank you. I love you."*
> – HO'OPONOPONO

Cherish quietude and time alone and choose to be in silence sometimes. God is the Infinite Truth abiding in the silence. Silence is the gateway to internal life, eternal life, and inner, infinite power. Silence is the temple of the Most High. There is peace, safety, wisdom, and infinite Love in silence. The quieter you become, the more you can hear. Being comfortable being alone is being powerful.

*"One of the best lessons you can learn in life
is to master how to remain calm.
Calmness is a superpower."*
– Bruce Lee

Spending more time in Nature, which is Living Intelligence strengthens will power. Move, exercise, and sweat every day. Smile more often and laugh every day.

*"Our body is our greatest ally.
It has access to all the wisdom and power
in the Universe, for it is syntropy itself.
Our divine key to access all of this is our will."*
– Souvereign

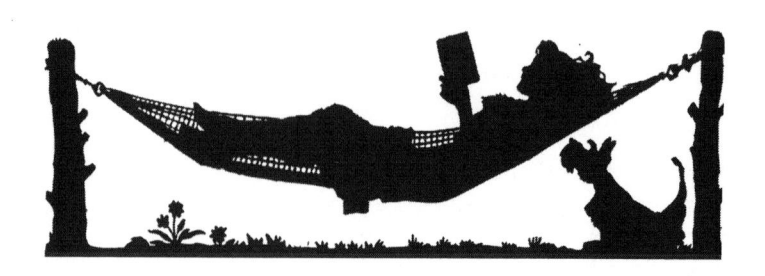

# WHAT TO AVOID

Avoid imposing your will and beliefs upon others. Energy is wasted trying to change and control others.

Avoid allowing the external/outside world to control you. It is empowering to choose to respond rather than react to outer circumstances. Breathe. Count to 10. Practice the pause. Take a time out. Choose to react in a constructive or neutral way to every event in Life. By not acting recklessly, life force energy is preserved. Do not allow words or the choices of others to provoke a reaction or to cause pain. How a person treats you reflects that person's self-love and emotional maturity. Go beyond acceptance and rejection. Do not waste time, energy, or money following fashions and trends for they soon lose their glamour. Create your own personal style.

Avoid following orders. Following orders means doing what you are told to do without judging for yourself whether the action is right or wrong, moral or immoral. Order followers are the biggest obstacle to the freedom of Humanity. Order followers keep the system of slavery in place, not those who give the orders. Order followers receive full karmic consequences. Order followers have no conscience, integrity, courage, or power.[67] "I am following orders," must never be an excuse for violating the free will of others, doing harm, or transgressing Natural Law. Nazism,

---

[67] Order-followers include members of police and military forces, prison staff, politicians, lobbyists, government employees, teachers in public education, doctors, nurses, members of cults/religions/political parties, mainstream media, and wage and debt slaves.

communism, fascism, socialism, and totalitarianism are only possible if people follow orders. Practice civil disobedience. In the words of Mexican revolutionary Emiliano Zapata, "It is infinitely more empowering to die on one's feet than to live on one's knees."

> *"You assist an evil system most effectively by obeying its orders and decrees. Allegiance to it means partaking of the evil. A good person will resist an evil system with his or her whole soul."*
> – Mahatma Gandhi

Avoid self-deprecation. Be gentle and compassionate with oneself. Participating in this earthly experiment of living in separation from All That Is at this time of shifting paradigms and transfiguration of our species is extremely challenging. No negative self-talk. There are no mistakes, only learning opportunities. Learn and integrate the lessons and move on.

> *"Don't be so tough on yourself about past mistakes, about missed opportunities, about trusting the advice of others over your own intuition. Make amends where you can. Forgive yourself for not knowing better before you knew better, and realize that the lessons were needed and had to be learned firsthand.*
> *Be tougher on yourself with following through with your ideas, your plans, dreams, and goals, and staying committed to making the changes*

*you want to make to better yourself, your life, and your future."*
– Doe Zantamata

Avoid suppressing "negative" emotions. There is no bypassing the intense energies of anger, rage, sadness, grief, and fear. There is much to learn from emotions – messages, lessons, treasures, morals, and seeds of Truth. Emotion is energy in motion. Feeling emotions makes you human. Suppressing these emotions makes you physically and mentally ill. Expressing these emotions in ways that make others suffer in any way makes you inhuman. Allow emotions to flow through you. Ongoingly process, release, emote, vent to decrease fear, anxiety, guilt, shame, grief, sadness, frustration, rage, and anger, and return to balance. Transmute destructive emotions to constructive emotions or suffer from physical and/or mental illnesses. The feeling is the healing. Allow yourself to fully feel emotions in a way that harms no-one. All crying is healing. Crying frees the mind from sorrowful thoughts and heavy burdens. Be willing to feel uncomfortable, messy, and snotty. And to sound unhuman. Healing, change, and growth are not always easy, pretty, and comfortable.

*"Don't be afraid to cry.
It will free your mind of sorrowful thoughts."*
– Hopi saying

Anger, including righteous anger, is toxic, degenerative, and destructive to self and society. Anger creates ill health, depletes energy, accelerates aging, and creates an anti-social personality. An angry disposition harms the heart and interferes with energy generation and circulation. Anger, aggression, and impatience deplete Lifeforce energy. Peacefulness and patience build Lifeforce energy. Having a temper will destroy your health, your character, and your relationships. Never let anger get out of hand. Allowing anger to fester is a crime against Humanity. Make time to release and clear anger and rage (and trauma) regularly in ways that do no harm and balance is restored: Scream and cry into a pillow or a towel. Scream and rant alone in a car. Punch a punching bag. Smash a cardboard box. Exercise. Shake. Clean. Do yard work. Do breathwork. Externalize/verbalize thoughts and feelings in a safe, sacred space. Write down feelings and burn the pages. Putting pen to paper acts as a poultice. Visit a rage room or join a scream club. Yell into a hole in the ground. Give negative emotions to Earth for transmutation, and Earth gives back Love. Never prepare food, make life decisions, or breastfeed when angry.

Refuse to stay in any dark mental states. Avoid wallowing in depression. helplessness, despondency, hopelessness, despair, and suicidal ideation. These states of mind weaken us mentally and physically while strengthening the presence of evil on Earth. It is empowering to know that there is always light at the end of every tunnel, that everything changes, and that every situation will pass, leaving a gift and a lesson. Seeking answers to the question, "What is this person/situation/

experience teaching me?" is most beneficial. Everything happens for personal growth and evolution.

Avoid being incapacitated by fear. Face fears. Wisdom and power arise from identifying and overcoming fears. Replace fearful thoughts with better-feeling thoughts that are true, positive, empowering, and life-affirming. Act and do the right thing, despite fear and/or public opinion. Embrace immortality and act courageously. Only action creates change, not mouse-clicking or looking at screens, which are designed to capture our attention and energy.

***Your power ends where your fear begins.***

Avoid squandering the power of attention. Avoid being distracted. Avoid excessive thinking, excessive socializing, and excessive labor, which deplete the body of generative energy. Balance movement and rest. Break addictions to mental activity, overthinking, acquiring knowledge, and scheming. Abide in the stillness.

Avoid squandering mental energy, physical energy, and sexual energy, which happens through excessive ejaculation for men. Avoid wasting time, food, money, words, resources, and creative power. Break addictions to all activities that do not promote health, happiness, empowerment, or freedom. If one squanders personal power and Divine gifts, the flow of abundance and Grace will stop. One must prove oneself to be a trustworthy recipient of Divine power before wisdom, abundance, and Grace are bestowed and the mysteries of Life are revealed. Conserve, restore, and accumulate Lifeforce energy, because it is intricately linked to lifespan. When it is depleted, death of the physical body occurs.

Stop complaining, gossiping, arguing, and airing grievances, problems, physical ailments, and burdens, which deplete personal power. Stop overanalyzing oneself, other people, the newsfeed, politics, and the antics and agendas of the Old Order, which is being reduced to beggary and impotence. We will end the enslavement of Humanity by starving the parasites and their control systems of our attention and energy and focusing on co-creating New Earth by embodying Divine Love.

Avoid creating disharmony and drama. Stop passive-aggressive behaviors, like slamming doors and "The Silent Treatment." Stop seeking, participating in, and fueling conflicts. No bickering. Stop being a joy-destroying, mean, moody, unkind, selfish, controlling, attention-seeking, needy, greedy, helpless person. Avoid loneliness.

> *Just be a good human.*
> *Be humble. Be kind. Be grateful. Be of service.*
> *Radiate health, happiness, and peace.*
> *Spread joy, peace, and Love.*

Avoid giving power away to other people, organizations, religions, movements, causes, and influencers. Those who seek to vampirize human energy are known as Energy Vampires and Narcissists. They are everywhere – online and in person. Beware and be vigilant. Establish boundaries for protection. "No" is an immensely powerful word. "No Contact" is the most empowering strategy.

> *"When one person suffers from a delusion,*
> *it's called insanity.*
> *When many people suffer from a delusion,*
> *it's called a religion."*
> – Robert. M. Pirsig

Avoid seeking approval, attention, flattery, confirmation, validation, permission, and energy from others. All one needs is found within. Celebrate your uniqueness and love your individual, essential contribution to the whole of Life. No-one is more powerful, more integral, or more loved than you. Stop deferring to other people, comparing oneself, trying to please others, and caring about what others think or say. Caring what others think of you breeds mental illness and powerlessness. It is not possible to be powerful, happy, or free if one lives life based on other people's opinions and expectations..

Avoid toxic food, people, relationships, and environments. Avoid fearmongers, and news and information sources that escalate fears and confuscate, hide, and censor information that contradicts official narratives/lies. Avoid shirking responsibilities and duties.

# LOVE ALWAYS WINS.

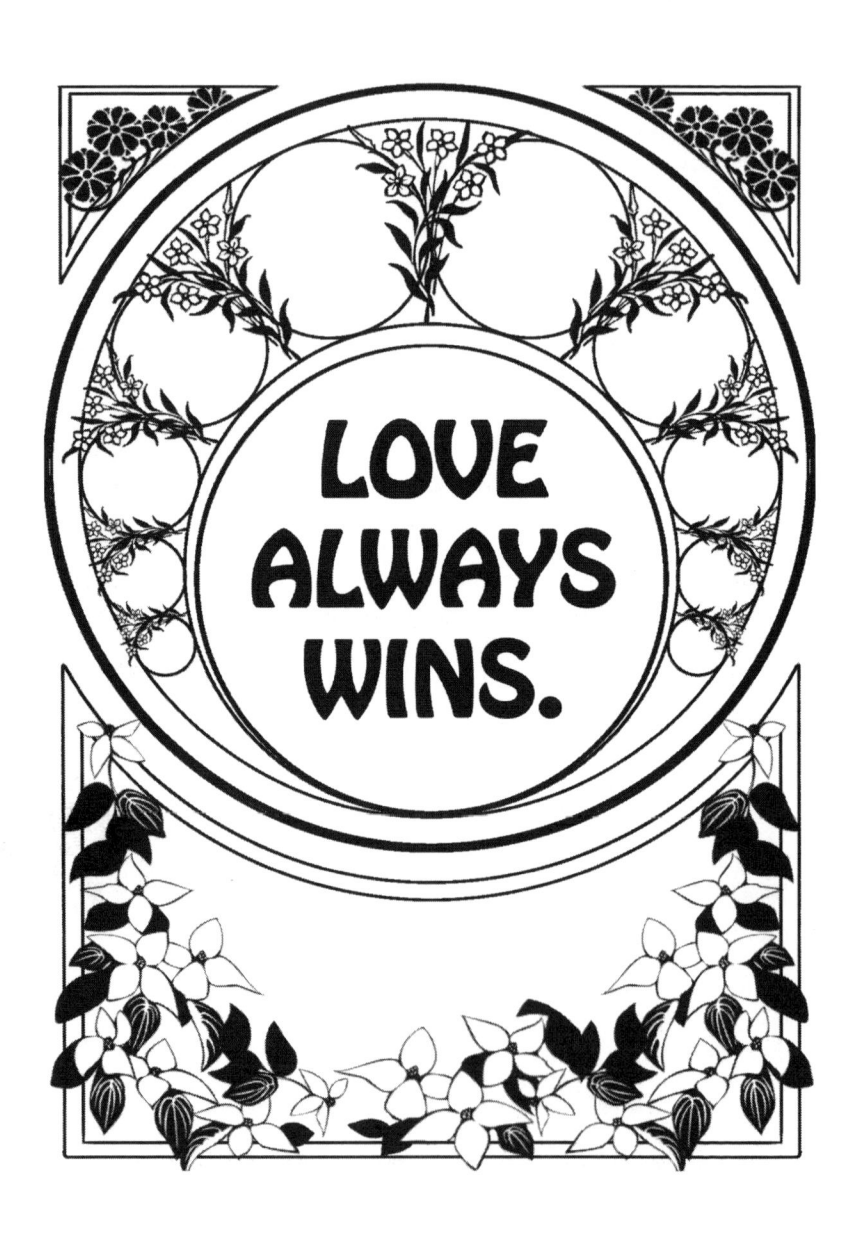

# INCREASING PHYSICAL POWER

**Our health is our supreme power.**

All indigenous wisdom traditions, shamanic traditions, ancient mystery schools, yogic traditions, marital arts schools, and ancient schools of medicine have principles, practices, techniques, tools, medicines, mantras, yantras. mudras, asanas, and teachings that align personal energy and anatomical geometry with Universal energy and sacred geometry to restore balance, improve health, and increase energy and personal power. Western/Rockefeller "medicine" is not medicine because it is unnatural, poisonous, profit-driven, puts profits over lives. and fails to take energy into account – which is the most important factor for understanding life, optimizing health, and living as a sovereign being. Choosing to learn from any of these ancient and sacred traditions can increase personal power and personal responsibility, for oneself and for one's energy.

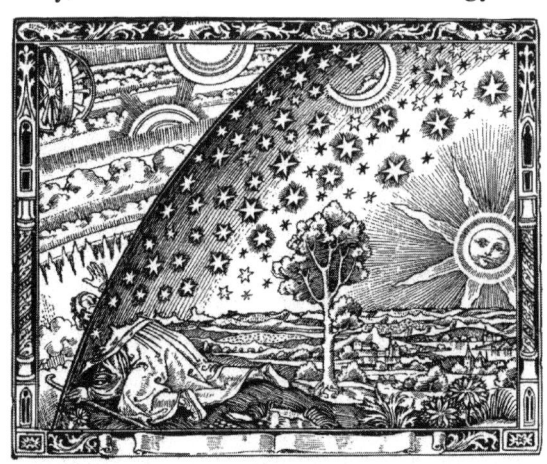

For example, meditating on the Sri Yantra (below) increases personal power.

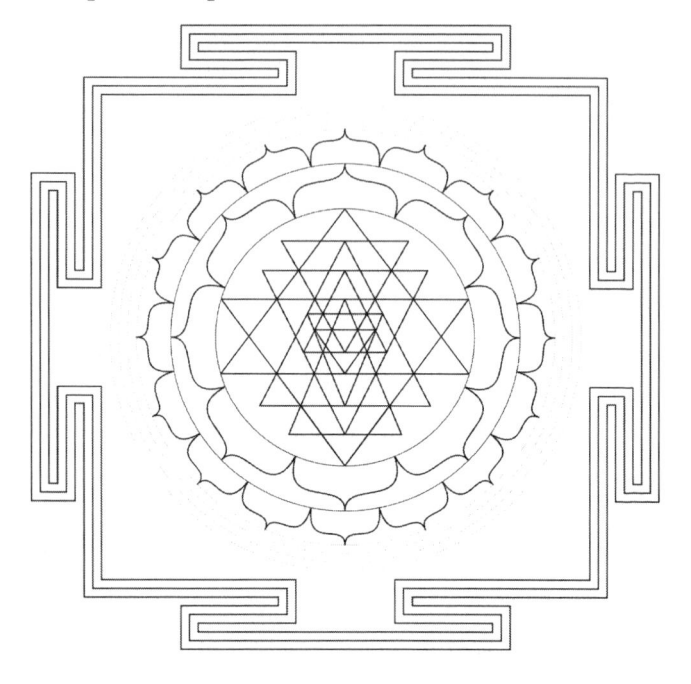

The most important principle underlying health, happiness, freedom, and personal power is to live in alignment with Natural Law – Cosmic Spiritual Law.

> ***Do no harm. Cause no loss.***
> ***Commit no fraud. Keep the peace.***
> ***Protect, preserve, and honor***
> ***all expressions of Life/Love/Light.***
> ***Do what leads to greater Love,***
> ***and what serves the highest good.***

Cherish the physical body. Preserve and protect Lifeforce energy. Protect the body from extreme heat, cold, dryness, and dampness. And from poisons and parasites. Avoid loud and dissonant music and noises, decaying smells, artificial lighting, and overly spicy foods, which disrupt inner balance and harmony. Rest when appropriate and act when necessary. Practice self-love and self-care. Cultivate a loving relationship with your physical body. Listen to intuition – the inner teacher – which speaks through sensations, imagery, visions, dreams, and symbols. Send Love and gratitude to every cell and all parts of your body, organs, and systems. Loving energy can be directed to any part of the body that needs healing.

Do any kind of physical activity to maintain cardiovascular fitness, strength, flexibility, and agility. Sweat. Stretch. Strengthen. Build core strength: Yoga. Pilates. Rebounding. Cycling. Squatting.[68] Dance alone and with others. Participate in Outdoor Adventure activities. A 20-minute daily walk in Nature is a life-changing practice. Taking a walk after a meal can be a beneficial practice.

Structural alignment of the physical body is essential for optimal well-being and empowerment. Alignment is the proper, natural positioning of the head, shoulders, spine, hips, knees, ankles, and feet so that they line up vertically with each other. When the body is aligned, movement is efficient, fluid, and pain-free, and we function in the most economical and powerful way. When the body is out of alignment, additional stress and strain is created on the body – joints, muscles,

---

[68] http://squateverywhere.com/

fascia, and bones. Being out of alignment puts one in a state of detriment and can lead to injuries, stiffness, discomfort, loss of energy, loss of strength, loss of confidence, kyphosis, and osteoporosis. It is easy for the body to move out of alignment from the pull of gravity, daily physical activities, repetitive movements, sports, birthing, childcare, and physical traumas. It is important to be properly aligned when sitting, standing, walking, jogging, climbing stairs, pushing, pulling, lifting, and carrying to reduce risk of damage and injury.

Structural alignment and good posture allow optimal flow of energy throughout the body, which is necessary for health, healing, and vitality. When there are obstructions to energy flow, dying sets in. When the body is aligned and relaxed, we receive optimal flow of Lifeforce energy throughout all energy channels and centers. When the physical body is in alignment, all organs, systems, and cells can function optimally. By standing tall, as if there is an invisible cord pulling upward from the top of the head, spine is long, feet firmly planted on the ground, and shoulders back and down, the flow of energy throughout the body is increased. Poor posture, slouching, slumping, and being out of structural alignment blocks the flow of Lifeforce energy. There are many ways to develop good posture, strength, and proper body use, and to realign the body and maintain balanced alignment: Tai Chi. Qi Gong. Yoga. Pilates. Eurythmy. Calisthenics. An osteopathic adjustment. A chiropractic adjustment. Structural Bodywork. Structural Integration. Rolfing. Massage therapy. Physical therapy. Acupuncture. Grounding. Walking.

> *"When we feel at home in our bodies,
> we feel at home in the world."*
> – Lama Rod Owens

Optimize brain health to achieve mental, physical, and planetary balance, and optimize personal power. Study nutrition. Personalize and optimize nutrition. Listen to intuition. Tune into the body and listen to what it is communicating. Is there pain, stiffness, numbness, heat, tingling, tension, or tears? What does it need? Food? Hydration? Rest? Emotional release? Exercise? A hug? Nature? Always listen to and follow intuitive information. Intuitive ability and personal power are increased every time intuitive information is heeded. It may be necessary to optimize health with nutritional supplements and superfoods because most humans and all chemically grown fruits and vegetables are severely depleted of nutrients, vitamins, cell salts, and Lifeforce energy.

Embrace a vegetarian or vegan lifestyle.[69] The purpose of food is to maintain and protect life. Ingesting anything that does not fulfill this purpose is not wise or advantageous. Eating factory-farmed meat at every meal destroys physical health and depletes personal power. Eating meat, meat products, and unnatural, denatured, and highly processed foods unnecessarily taxes the body, overburdens organs and tissues, and creates toxicity and inflammation, which is the underlying cause of most chronic diseases. Toxins from store

---

[69] https://feelingbetternaturally.love/writing/f/embracing-a-vegan-lifestyle

bought meat (and all unnatural, ingested substances) irritate nerves and glands, which lays the foundation for poor mental and physical health. Meat-eating creates acidity in the body, which is ideal for the growth of cancers. Excess consumption of meat causes damage to the heart. Graphene oxide, nanotechnologies, and other toxins have been found in meats. The meat industry is extremely cruel, environmentally destructive, satanic, and grossly unsustainable. All products are depleted and depleting in every way. Eating factory-farmed meat suppresses sensitivity and empathy, causes loss of emotional intelligence, and increases aggression. Not eating factory-farmed meat and not using cruelly derived products is best for personal and planetary health.

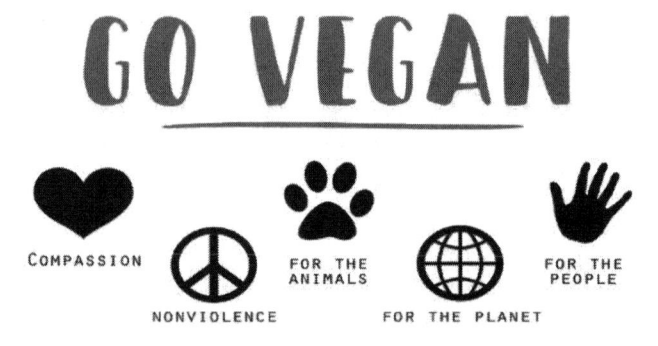

## GO VEGAN

**COMPASSION** — **NONVIOLENCE** — **FOR THE ANIMALS** — **FOR THE PLANET** — **FOR THE PEOPLE**

A plant-based diet is a more efficient, effective, beneficial, and humane way to receive optimal nutrition and nourishment. Eat natural, high-quality, organic, nutrient-dense, minimally-processed foods. Eat a wide range of organic, living, raw, and sun-ripened fruits and vegetables that are high in photonic/living Light. Light is information/knowledge. Knowledge is power. Applied knowledge is wisdom. Eat more fresh vegetables, fruits, greens, herbs, microgreens, avocados, coconut and coconut water, sprouted seeds, nuts, and sprouted grains. Tropical fruits have the most photonic energy. Vegetables are best raw, lightly steamed, baked, or roasted, rather than boiled. Overcooking destroys Lifeforce energy. Eat more dark green, leafy vegetables. Green leaves are what power gorillas (who share 98 per cent of our DNA), and are essential for muscle strength and overall health.[70]

Prioritize gut health. Gut health creates mental health. There is a vast community of trillions of microorganisms including bacteria, fungi, viruses, archaea, and protozoa that colonize the gut, which is known as the gut microbiome or microbiota. Gut flora aid digestion and nutrient absorption and protect against malnourishment and invasive pathogens. Microbes in the gut produce beneficial compounds like vitamins and anti-tumor/anti-inflammatory compounds. Gut bacteria produce neurochemicals, which communicate with the brain via the enteric nervous system and regulate basic physiological and cognitive functions. The gut produces more neurotransmitters than the brain. A healthy gut produces 90% of the serotonin produced by the body.

***"Serotonin plays a crucial role in developing our forebrain, the region of the neocortex where learning, spirituality, and the higher emotions, such as love and altruism can be experienced. Serotonin also enhances the growth of neurons***

---

[70] Edith Cowan University: *New Research Finds Green Leafy Vegetables Essential for Muscle Strength*. www.scitechdaily.com, 24 March 2021. https://scitechdaily.com/new-research-finds-green-leafy-vegetables-essential-for-muscle-strength/

> *in the region of the brain that enables us to have new experiences – the hippocampus."*
> – ALBERTO VILLOLDO [71]

The human brain and the community of microorganisms in the gut have co-evolved to optimize the health and well-being of the human being. There is symbiosis between the brain and the gut. A flourishing microbial ecosystem in the gut plays a foundational role in our health and well-being. A flourishing gut microbiome is necessary for optimal health and personal power.

> *"Many of the diseases of modern living begin in the gut, and disturbances in the colony of microorganisms in the gut affect the functioning of the brain."*
> – ALBERTO VILLOLDO[72]

Dysbiosis, an imbalanced microbiome, is easily caused by modern living – consuming highly processed and junk foods, alcohol, refined sugars, refined oils, glyphosate, and other toxins in non-organic products, chemically grown grains, GMOs, synthetic and lab-grown substances, and hormones in non-organic meat. Antibiotics, vaccines, immunizations, flu shots, and many pharmaceutical and over-the-counter drugs destroy the gut microbiome. Environmental toxins, unhealthy

---

[71] Villoldo, Alberto. *Grow A New Body: How Spirit and Power Plant Nutrients Can Transform Your Health*. Hay House Inc, USA, 2019.

[72] ib. id.

lifestyle choices, stress, anxiety, and fear create dysbiosis.

Symptoms of dysbiosis include stomach pain, bloating, gas, fatigue, joint pain, allergies, skin irritations, sleep disturbances, food intolerances, brain fog, anxiety, and mood swings. Dysbiosis leads to serious health problems, including systemic inflammation, obesity, cancers, autoimmune disorders, hormonal imbalance, low immunity, intestinal disorders (diarrhea, constipation, irritable bowel syndrome, leaky gut, gluten intolerance, colorectal cancer), heart and other cardiovascular disorders (coronary artery disease, atherosclerosis, high blood pressure), and metabolic disorders (Type 2 diabetes). Brain disorders (Dementia, Alzheimer's disease, Parkinson's disease, Autism, ADHD), and mental health and mood disorders (depression, anxiety, panic attacks, psychoses, and schizophrenia) may arise as a result of dysbiosis.[73]

To support a healthy gut microbiome, it is necessary to address and avoid causes of dysbiosis. Stop ingesting unnatural and toxic substances and liquids. Recolonize and repair an imbalanced gut microbiome with probiotics, prebiotics, and fermented foods.[74] Fermented foods have benefits that

---

[73] Remmick, S. *How the Microbiome Controls Your Health.* Life Extension Magazine, June 2018. https://www.lifeextension.com/Magazine/2018/6/Role-Of-Microbiome-In-Whole-Body-Health/Page-01

[74] Fermented and cultured foods and drinks that support gut health include sauerkraut, kimchi, kefir, pickled vegetables, miso, tamari, tempeh, cultured condiments (natto, for example), kombucha, jun, tepaches, tejuinos, and unpasteurized apple cider vinegar. Foods made from coconut, including unsweetened coconut yogurt, coconut oil, and MCT (medium-chain triglyceride) oil derived from coconut oil promote gut health.

can be increased by prayers and intentions. These colonies of microorganisms in our gut and in fermented foods are intelligent lifeforms that can work in synergy with humans and respond when asked and appreciated. For this reason, making, thanking, and ingesting fermented foods optimizes their benefits. Re-establishing and maintaining a healthy gut takes time and effort. It is beneficial to practice relaxation.

Love is the most important factor in receiving optimal nutrition from what we eat. A true understanding of the relationship between love and food will revolutionize health. Love instructs food as to how to best nourish the body. Express gratitude for food. Grow and prepare food with love. Blessing food and those who grew, transported, and prepared it increases its potency. For optimal nutrition, strengthen your heart. A strong, fiercely loving heart establishes a higher frequency for bodily functions and promotes more efficient energy utilization. When the frequency of the body is Divine Love, it can manufacture all it needs without support or compensation. A loving heart facilitates the innate ability to manufacture vitamins through the replication of mineral frequencies. The lower frequency of the heart leaves us under supplied with self-made nutrients and unable to manufacture other substances and sacred secretions that will support our health and our transition to living in New Earth. Eat slowly and mindfully and chew thoroughly to extract maximum energy and nourishment.

Certain plants, known as adaptogens, strengthen our ability to adapt to psychological, physical, and environmental stressors. These plants contain substances that have balancing, restorative, and overall toning effects. Adaptogens can also improve immune function, support weight management, increase physical endurance and mental focus, reduce the discomfort of poor health, and support a balanced mood. Adaptogens increase our Lifeforce energy and promote longevity. Many plants function as adaptogens - power plants.[75]

Water is life and water is alive. Dr Masaru Emoto demonstrated that water responds to consciousness.[76] Thoughts change the nature of water. Given that the human body is mostly water, we benefit from thinking positive thoughts, and we are sickened by thinking negative thoughts. Stay hydrated by drinking pure, alkaline, non-fluoridated, non-chlorinated water. Drinking naturally structured water and

---

[75] Adaptogens include Ginger (*Zingiber officinale*), Kava Kava (*Piper methysticum*), Korean Ginseng (*Panax ginseng*), American Ginseng (*Panax quinquefolius*), Siberian ginseng (*Eleutherococcus senticosus*), Golden Root (*Rhodiola rosea*), Tibetan Rhodiola (*Rhodiola sacra*), Brazilian Ginseng/Suma (*Pfaffia paniculate*), Ashwagandha (*Withania somnifera*), Acai Berries (*Euterpe oleracea*), Astragalus Root (*A. membranaceus*), Tulsi/Holy Basil (*Ocimum sanctum*), Licorice Root (*Glycyrrhiza glabra*), *Schizandra chinesis*, Jiaogulan (*Gynostemma*), Chaga mushroom (Inonotus obliquus) Reishi mushroom (*Ganoderma lucidum*), Shiitake mushroom (*Lentinula edodes*), Maitake mushroom (*Grifolia frondosa*), *Cordyceps sinensis*, Goji Berries (*Lycium*), Rosemary (*Rosamarinus officinalis*), Aloe Vera, Maca (*Lepidium meyenii*), Bacopa Monnieri, Gotu Kola (*Centella asiatica*), Elderberry (*Sambucus nigra*), Bilberry (*Vaccinium myrtillus*), Turmeric (*Curcuma longa*), Amla (*Phyllanthus emblica*), *Moringa oleifera*, *Cannabis sativa*, *C. indica*, *C. ruderalis*, Spirulina (*Arthrospira*), Chlorella (*Chlorella vulgaris*), Wheatgrass (*Triticum aestivum*) and Barleygrass (*Hordeum vulgare*), and Shilajit. https://www.globalhealingcenter.com/natural-health/what-are-adaptogens/https://www.wisewomanschool.com/p/adaptogens-herbs-for-energy-longevity-and-optimum-health

[76] Emoto, M. *The Hidden Messages in Water*. Beyond Words Publishing Inc. Oregon, USA. 2004

water that has been through a vortex or programmed with a crystal is optimal. Water connects us with our ancestors and intensifies our prayers. Water can be infused by prayers to optimize health, well-being, and personal power. Drinking prayer-infused water is highly beneficial.

De-tox and e-tox[77] daily. Undertake cleanses from physical, emotional, spiritual, electromagnetic, vibrational, and environmental toxicity. Use water, crystals, Orgone, smudging, essential oils, herbs, green leaves, sweating, fasting, juicing, enemas, colonics, breathwork, bodywork, and energy work. Use Nature, sunlight, sounds, silence, entheogens, and meditation.

**Detoxify to be intoxicated by the Divine.**

Breathing with intention can increase personal power. When you can control your breath, you can control your life. When you change the way you breath, you change your reality because breathing is alchemy. There are countless breathing techniques that can be practiced to increase personal power. Deep, relaxed, slow, rhythmic, full-belly breathing is far more beneficial and empowering than shallow, upper chest breathing. Shallow breathing reduces air flow, which stimulates the sympathetic nervous system and triggers a stress response in the body. Cortisol, the stress hormone, floods the body, taxes the adrenal glands, and negatively

---

[77] e-tox: Disconnecting and living free from electronic devices for extended periods of time.

# Smudging Prayer

May your hands be cleansed,
that they create beautiful things.

May your feet be cleansed,
that they might take you where you most need to be.

May your heart be cleansed,
that you might hear its message clearly.

May your throat be cleansed,
that you may speak rightly when words are needed.

May your eyes be cleansed,
that you may see the sign and wonders of this world.

May this person and space be washed clean
by the smoke of these fragrant plants.

And may that same smoke carry our paryers
spiralling to the heavens.

Please and Thank You.

impacts the whole body. Practicing and establishing correct, natural, deep breathing promotes optimal physical health, physical energy, mental power, emotional balance, self-control, clear-sightedness, happiness, inner peace, and spiritual growth. By holding the intention that each inbreath brings Lifeforce energy, healing energy, power, and whatever else is needed for optimal health, one can increase personal power, health, and well-being. Intend that all that no longer serves one's highest good is released on the outbreath. Avoid mouth breathing.

> *"Life is the emergence of breath.*
> *When breath emerges, there is life.*
> *When breath stops, there is death.*
> *Life and death are a matter of the*
> *appearance and disappearance of breath."*
> — Eva Wong[78]

In addition to breathing though the nose and mouth, we can breathe in and out through every pore, every chakra,[79] the heart, and every organ, including our sexual organs. Sexual organs concentrate the greatest amount of vital force energy and are the most powerful battery in the human system.

---

[78] YouTube: *Being Taoist: Wisdom for Living a Balanced Life by Eva Wong* [*FULL AUDIOBOOK | REMASTERED AUDIO*]. Spiritual Audiobooks, 2 March 2021. https://www.youtube.com/watch?v=eOmuIBEEyMk

[79] Understanding the chakra system is essential for unlocking keys to health, happiness, and power. The Third Chakra is our power center, our Solar Plexus, the seat of our will. Breathing golden energy into this chakra will increase personal power. See the work of Mantak Chia.

Breathing energy into the sexual organs strengthens and tones them, which strengthens us mentally, physically, and morally. One of the most powerful practices for increasing personal power for women is to breathe Earth energy in and out through the yoni/vagina.[80]

Smile and laugh more often. Choose to induce laughter in self and others. Radiate positivity and optimism as much as possible. We are manifesting New Earth by emanating joy, peace, loving kindness, and Love/Light.

***The biggest leap in frequency
comes when you laugh.***

Get quality sleep. Essential detoxification, repair, and rejuvenation processes take place in the brain during sleep. Sleep connects us with Infinite Intelligence, where all potentialities exist. Create sleep hygiene by going to bed before you are tired in a peaceful state of mind and in a dark, slightly cool room. Oversleeping and sleep deprivation weaken us, mentally and physically. A nap is empowering. A morning devotional ritual is empowering. Upon awakening, give thanks for life, for the opportunity to serve God for another day, and visualize the day as you would like it to unfold. Bless everyone and everything. Greet and meet every day with positive expectancy.

Stay clean and groomed. Wear clean clothes. Live in a

---

[75] Another powerful practice for women to connect with the Earth and receive Earth energy is to offer menstrual blood to the Earth every moon cycle.

clean, uncluttered space. Protect oneself from physical, emotional, and spiritual harm, and from environmental and electromagnetic toxicity. Ongoingly release anxiety, tension, and stress. Practice relaxation. When the body is relaxed, energy flows freely without obstruction and life energy is preserved. Give yourself a foot massage. Lovingly apply pure, natural oils. Perform all acts of self-care with deep love and reverence for the body, as it is a sacred vehicle for soul evolution.

Appreciate and savor Life through all the senses. Slow down and make time to savor food, scents, sensations, and sunsets. Stop and smell the roses. Listen to high vibrational music, frequencies, and sounds of Nature. Appreciate sacred art and texts, ecstatic poetry, and indigenous mythology to stimulate higher response centers, raise one's vibrational frequency, expand consciousness, and increase personal power.

Develop latent, innate gifts – intuition, psychic abilities, extrasensory perceptions, telepathy, telekinesis, clairaudience. clairvoyance, claircognizance, remote viewing, lucid dreaming, timeline traveling, psychometry,[81] and channeling.[82]

Practice raising Chrism every month – the Sacred Secretion or Oil of Christ. There are sacred secretions produced by the body that raise consciousness, activate multidimensionality, and increase personal power. Knowledge of this exquisite practice has been occulted because it is knowledge of

---

[81] Reading the history of inanimate objects.

[82] Energetic connection and communication with unseen intelligences.

infinite power, rejuvenation, and immortality. This physical, metaphysical, and astrological activation releases supernatural, superhuman energy that informs and transforms us, and activates our full potential. It brings physiological renewal and has been used by our ancestors to live for hundreds, even thousands, of years – the true fountain of youth and the elixir of life.[83]

> *"When certain areas of the brain are stimulated by the secret process of the Mysteries, the consciousness of man is extended, and he is permitted to behold the Immortals and enter into the presence of superior gods."*
> – BOOK OF THOTH[84]

Go outdoors to be immersed in Nature as often as possible. Earth is alive and always offering all that sustains Life. Breathe fresh, tree-filtered air and feel the sun and wind on your skin. Frequent exposure to Nature is imperative for optimal mental and physical health. Without health, one is powerless. Without regular and extended time in Nature, mental and physical illnesses will arise and persist. Visit backyards, parks, gardens,

---

[83] Research "Sacred Secretion," "Chrism," and "Sacred Oil of Christ." https://universaltruthschool.com/syncretism/raising-the-chrism/

[84] Hall, M.P. *The Secret Teachings of All Ages*, H.S. Crocker Co., Inc., San Francisco, USA. 1928.
https://www.cia.gov/library/abbottabad-compound/E4/
E4AAFF6DAF6863F459A8B4E52DFB9FF4_Manly.P.Hall_The.Secret.Teachings.of.All.Ages.pdf

botanical gardens, community gardens, healing gardens,[85] rooftop gardens, tree-lined streets, florists, nurseries, farms, forests, deserts, mountains, beaches, lakes, streams, rivers, and wilderness.

Earth is a living being who responds to consciousness, mutualism, and physical contact. Earth benefits as much from love, appreciation, and direct contact with us as we do from Her. Send Love, Light, reverence, and gratitude to the Earth and receive Life Force energy, power, nurture, nourishment, positive electrons, and negative ions – antioxidants that destroy free radicals and reduce inflammation. Immediate benefits of being in Nature include reduced anxiety, increased relaxation, and improved mood. As time spent in Nature increases, extraordinary benefits to physical and psychological well-being are reported, including healing, radical remission, spontaneous awakening, and wisdom.[86] Continue to visit the same place in Nature and become the silent observer, the student, the lover, and the beloved. Nature is always communicating, and it is prudent to listen. Strengthen personal connection to Earth by falling in love with the natural world. Deepen the connection to Nature by feeling gratitude as a constant practice. Appreciate beauty everywhere – in the microcosm and the macrocosm.

---

[85] DiLonardo, M.J., *Borrowing the Power of a Healing Garden*, 24 March 2021. https://www.treehugger.com/borrowing-power-healing-gardens-5117057

[86] YouTube: *The Grounded*, Earthing, 10 September 2015. https://www.youtube.com/watch?v=cRWoXO2xWn4

***When you realize HEART is an anagram of
EARTH, it all makes sense.***

Give back for all that is given. Give more than you receive. Never take without asking or receive without expressing gratitude. Make offerings of water, flowers, fruits, incense, tears, blood, urine, sweat, and self. Follow the moon cycle. Dance under the stars. Make Love on the Earth. Drink rainwater and spring water. Swim/dip your toes in streams, lakes, rivers, hot springs, the ocean. Go on a picnic. Go biking, hiking, and camping. Take only photos and leave no trace. Pick up trash wherever you go. The more we give of ourselves to Earth and to Life itself, the more Life gives to us. This is how we heal, strengthen, enlighten, and empower ourselves to live as sovereign beings then help others to do the same. This is the Great Work we are here to do.

***"The human being, indeed the well-being of all creatures, depends on a positive connection with Nature, and specifically with untrammeled wilderness. Wilderness, the freedom of the natural world, calls humankind back to the enduring sanity and intelligence of wild things."***
– Wayne Teasdale

Bring more plants and flowers indoors. Plants filter air, improve mood, and facilitate healing and well-being. Pictures and videos of plants/Nature are also beneficial. Grow a garden. Grow at least some edible plants: Sprouts. Herbs. Greens.

Microgreens. Mushrooms from a *Grow Fungi at Home* kit. Feed and infuse plants with love and prayers and the plants will become personalized medicine to optimize health.

> *"The Nature around us and the nature within us form together a common communion, and when 'the within' and 'the without' are in harmony, man is well. When the nature in him and the nature around him have formed a powerful camaraderie of purpose, that individual is in harmony. And being in harmony, he is capable of the greatest achievements of which man is capable. Man can never be happy until he uses the powers he possesses as they were intended to be used to serve the common good."*
> – MANLY P. HALL[87]

Remain grounded, connected to Earth energy, and tapped into primal power and the never-ending, ever-present river of Life. Earth is the battery from which we recharge and recalibrate. Earth is covered by a sea of the electrons, which must be directly accessed to maintain health, homeostasis, strength, and vitality.[88]

---

[87] YouTube: *Manly P. Hall: Healing Power of Nature: Thoreau's Walden (remastered)*, Manly Hall Society. 7 March 2021. https://www.youtube.com/watch?v=wZ-_D9cUEXI&t=4663s.

[88] Ober, C., Sinatra, S., T, & Zucker, M. *Grounding: The Most Important Health Discovery Ever*. Basic Health Publications Inc. USA 2014.
YouTube: *The Grounded*. Earthing. 10 September 2015.
https://www.youtube.com/watch?v=cRWoXO2xWn4

***We need to be grounded to stand our ground,
and it is time to stand our ground.
It is time to be united by
our love for Truth and Freedom.***

To be grounded, make Earthing a daily practice - skin to Earth. Bare feet on Earth as often as possible for as long as possible. Lie on the Earth. Touch and hug trees, rocks, plants, flowers, crystals, other grounded people, and grounded animals (outdoor pets and farm animals). Concrete and bricks conduct Earth energy and promote Earthing. Earthing is the primary treatment for chronic and degenerative diseases, chronic stress, inflammation, pain, sleep disorders, depression, PTSD, and other imbalances. Earthing promotes relaxation and reduces blood viscosity, a major factor in cardiovascular disease. Modern life prevents connection to Earth energy, and most people are severely depleted, suffering unnecessarily, and missing out on innumerable benefits Earth is always offering.

***Imagine roots of Light
extending from the soles
of the feet, deep down into
Earth. Imagine branches
of Light extending from
the top of the head into
the Cosmos.***

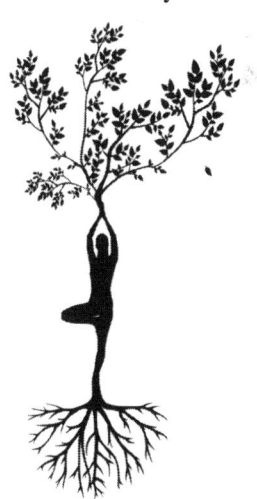

Wear shoes with soles made of natural materials. Eat root vegetables. Wear natural fibers and essential oils. Use natural lighting. Children, indoor pets, and plants also need to be grounded. To be healthy, children need to be outdoors for at least 4-6 hours daily.

Go barefoot as much as possible. Moving through life with bare feet increases groundedness, resilience, awareness, gratefulness, vitality, and personal power. Going barefoot balances our electrical/nervous circuitry, both brain hemispheres, and masculine and feminine energies, which optimizes energy flow to and throughout the body. Walking barefoot requires mindfulness and focus on the path with no distractions. With bare feet, it is not possible to move forward without being fully present, taking utmost care, and being aware of each footfall. It is beneficial to remove constrictions on the feet, which are as sensitive and as endowed with nerve endings and creative energy meridians as our hands. Activating the feet activates more cognitive power, higher consciousness, ancient DNA codes, creative power, strength, and a deep reverence for Life. Personal power increases as the ability to perceive more of reality increases, which happens when our feet are not always encased in shoes and disconnected from Earth. Choose natural-soled shoes that do not insulate one from Life or restrict the ability to move through the world as a balanced, grounded, intuitive, empowered human being. Daily Earthing engenders profound relationships with Earth, Nature, and Source. The more Earthing you do, the better you will feel.

> *"Walk as if you are kissing the Earth with your feet."*
> – Thich Nhat Hanh

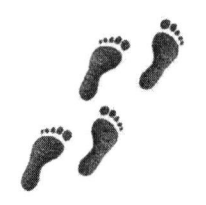

There are grounding technologies that can be used when access to Earth energy is not possible, including crystals, rocks, Orgone,[89] essential oils, and foods that grow underground like root vegetables. There are grounding devices for people, pets, homes, offices, and vehicles. Crystals are ever-spouting fountains of information and power, intelligent conduits and amplifiers of Lifeforce energy, and tools for balancing and healing – each with a unique signature and effect. Crystals remember, store, and provide information. There are crystals for empowerment, protection, grounding, balancing, amplifying, clearing, and upliftment, which can be worn and carried.

Go outdoors more often and get into sunlight. This is imperative. Sunlight is Life force energy, and most people are dangerously depleted after years on lockdown and imprisoned at home Sunlight is the highest and most essential information available to us while we are embodied. Sunlight is the consciousness of freedom. Fill yourself with sunlight at every opportunity – physically and metaphysically. Spending most of the time indoors, under artificial lighting, breathing carcinogenic air, and deprived of sunlight and Nature makes people extremely physically and mentally ill. We need sunlight on our skin and in our eyes for optimal health and

---

[89] Orgone energy is also known as prana, chi, or universal energy. Orgone energy can be accumulated and generated by layering organic and inorganic materials that harness and amplify this vital Lifeforce energy.

well-being. Receiving sunlight is the easiest and fastest way to raise the frequency of the body so it can perform optimally. The body chemically responds and begins to manufacture high-frequency nutrients that cannot be produced when the frequency/energy level of the body is low. It is beneficial to receive at least 20 minutes of sunlight on bare skin daily. No sunscreen. No overexposure. After 20 minutes in sunlight, the body releases 200 antimicrobials that fight pathogens and parasites. Wait to shower at least an hour after sun exposure so Vitamin D can be manufactured in the skin.

Fearing the Sun is fearing Life, itself. Instilling fear of looking at the Sun and being in sunlight has severely sickened, weakened, and disempowered human beings. It is evil genius to convince humans that the source of Life on Earth should be feared. Nothing could be more disempowering. Developing a loving relationship with the Sun is all-empowering and life changing. Sungazing is the easiest and most effective way to connect with the Sun, Prime Creator, and absolute Truth. Harmonic resonance with the Sun is created by daily sungazing, which will heal us at the deepest level and attract whatever is needed for soul evolution. One absorbs and accumulates the purifying power of the Sun, which burns away the illusions of earthly life. Sungazing will expedite expansion of perception and evolution of consciousness. This free and simple practice is the optimal way to improve the experience of each day and to increase vitality, creativity, courage, clarity, perseverance, personal power, and sleep quality.

**With bare feet on the earth, gaze gently at the Sun as it rises and sets.**

***Breathe deeply, relax, and receive.
Give thanks.***

Daily sungazing is the most powerful healing and transformational soul evolutionary practice available. Energy from the Sun can be directed to energize, revitalize, rejuvenate, and heal mind and body. And Earth and Humanity. There are options for indoor lighting and Light therapies that provide health benefits, such as improved mood, focus, relaxation, and mental clarity.[90]

Align with and strengthen connections with other sources of power in Nature. Energy flows where attention goes, so whatever you put your focus on exchanges energy with you in accordance with your intentions, integrity, and agreements. Discernment is essential. Countless benevolent beings and intelligences are waiting to connect, to exchange information and energy, to teach, to co-create, and to participate in our evolutionary journey: the elemental forces of Nature, Nature spirits, Earth, Air, Fire, Water, and Ether; the Four Directions; the planets, Sun and Moon, and other celestial bodies; all beings of Love and Light; and Infinite Intelligence. The all-powerful force of Nature is around you, with you, and in you, loving and empowering you. Drink deeply at every oppurtunity.

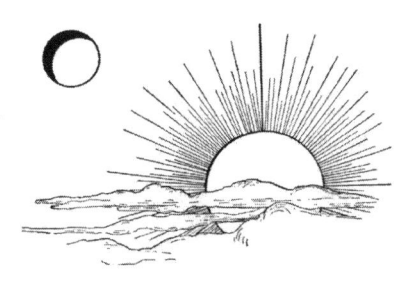

---

[90] Borchard, T. *6 Types of Light Therapy for Seasonal Depression*. www.everydayhealth.com 29 September 2016 https://www.everydayhealth.com/columns/therese-borchard-sanity-break/types-of-light-therapy-to-treat-seasonal-depression/

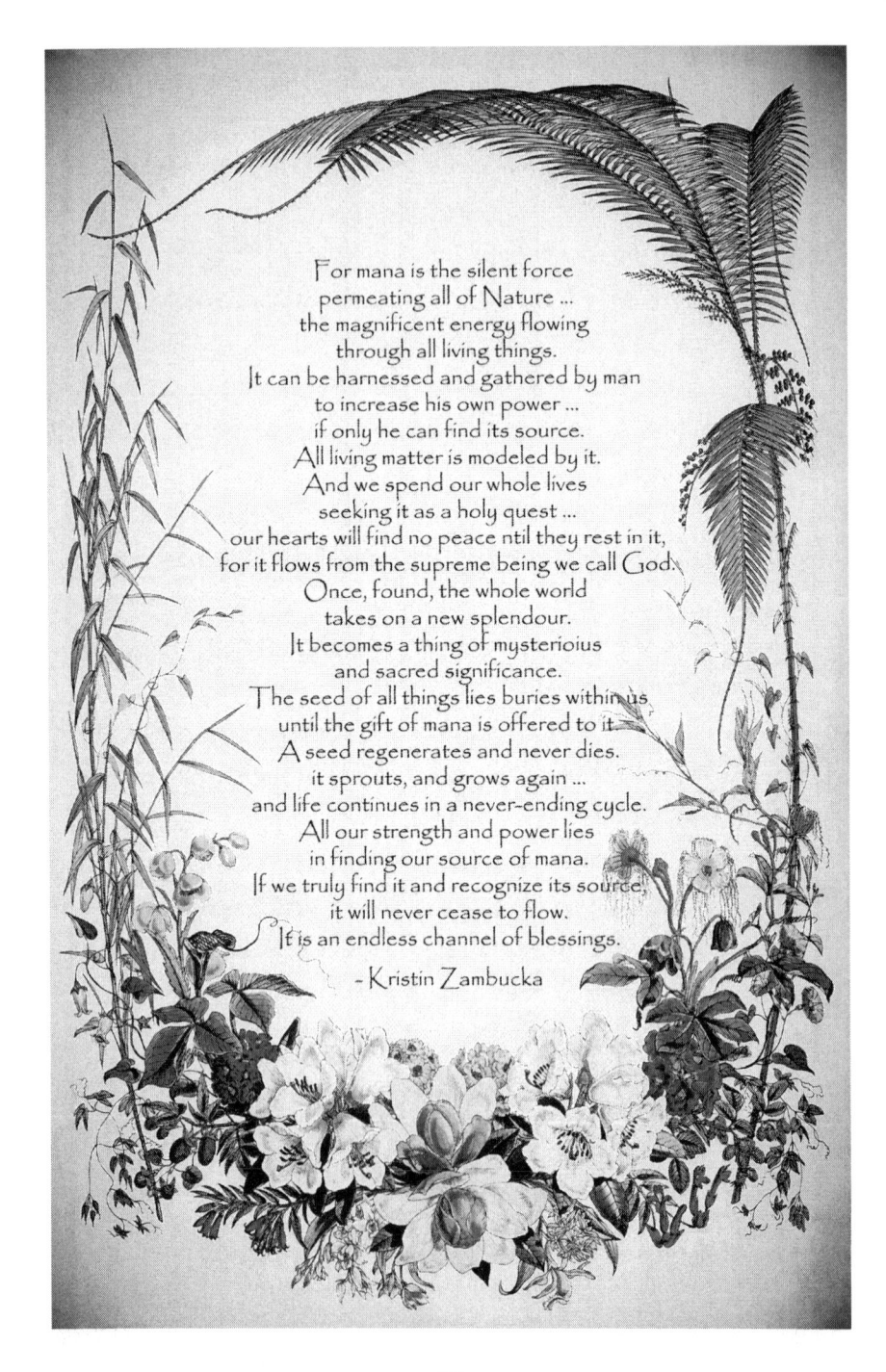

For mana is the silent force
permeating all of Nature ...
the magnificent energy flowing
through all living things.
It can be harnessed and gathered by man
to increase his own power ...
if only he can find its source.
All living matter is modeled by it.
And we spend our whole lives
seeking it as a holy quest ...
our hearts will find no peace ntil they rest in it,
for it flows from the supreme being we call God.
Once, found, the whole world
takes on a new splendour.
It becomes a thing of mysterioius
and sacred significance.
The seed of all things lies buries within us
until the gift of mana is offered to it.
A seed regenerates and never dies.
it sprouts, and grows again ...
and life continues in a never-ending cycle.
All our strength and power lies
in finding our source of mana.
If we truly find it and recognize its source,
it will never cease to flow.
It is an endless channel of blessings.

— Kristin Zambucka

***From Atman did space come into being:***
***from space, air;***
***from air, fire;***
***from fire, the waters;***
***from the waters, the earth;***
***from the earth, plants;***
***from the plants, food;***
***and from food, man."***
— Taittiriya Upanisad

Moongaze. Stargaze. Star Walk.[91] Cloud watch. Read the love letters sent by the wind, the rain, the sun, the Earth, and the Cosmos. Watch birds. Watch animals. Listen to the sounds of Nature: Rain. Ocean, Jungle. Birdsong. Windsong. Whalesong. Feel imbued by uplifting music, harmonious frequencies, and binaural beats. Feel as free as a bird. As fluid as water. As grounded as a tree. As solid as a rock. As energized as lightning. As fierce as Mars. As brilliant as the Sun. As disciplined as Saturn. As benevolent as Gaia. As loving as God.

Consider Entheogens.[92] There is consciousness within all

---

[91] A walk by starlight and moonlight.

[92] Entheogens include: Cannabis, THC (Tetrahydrocannabinol), Tobacco (*genus Nicotiana*), Psilocybin (genus *Psilocybe*), DMT (N, N-Dimethyltryptamine), Ayahauasca (*Banisteriopsis caapi*), *Salvia divinorum*, Peyote (*Lophophora williamsii*), San Pedro cactus/Huachuma ( *Echinopsis pachanoi*), Kava Kava (*Piper methysticum*), Iboga (*Tapernanthe iboga*), Kratom (*Mitragyna speciosa*), kanna (canna; *Mesembryanthemum expansum L. Sceletuim*), Monoatomic Gold (ormus), Nutmeg (*Myristica fragrans houtt*), Cacao (*Therobroma cacao*), Changa (a DMT-infused smoking blend of herbs),

things, and consciousness is always communicating. There are sacred plant medicines and other substances that expand consciousness, dissolve cultural indoctrination, correct perception, and connect one with God, with other higher intelligences, and with allies. Listen for their call. It is empowering to work with plant and other non-human allies to free the shackles from the subconscious mind, liberate and explore consciousness, and heal at the deepest level. Always make the practice sacred. Be reverent, be respectful, be grateful, and be sure to optimize (mind)set and setting.

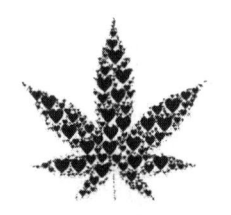

> ***You get the trip you need, which may not be the trip you want.***

It is empowering to visit megaliths, sacred sites, power places, energy vortexes, ley lines, and wilderness. Climb trees and mountains. Stand by the ocean, a waterfall, the confluence of rivers, and under the stars and the full moon. Sleep on the earth, in a tent, on a rooftop. Light and sit by a fire. Go on a pilgrimage. A Vision Quest. A Vigil. A retreat. A Shamanic journey.

The human body is a microcosm of the macrocosm of Heaven and Earth, and it is patterned after the Laws of the Universe. Follow and align with the cycles and energies of Nature – the waxing and waning of the sun and the moon, and

---

MDMA (3,4 -methylenedioxymethamphetamine), and LSD (Lysergic acid diethylamide).

the cycles and rhythms of the seasons and the stars. Follow the natural way. Sleep when it is dark. Rise with the sun. Eat seasonal fruits and vegetables. Sow seeds and start new ventures at the new moon. Harvest at the full moon. Renew yourself with the cycles of the seasons. Retreat, rest, and regenerate in Winter, and extend energy outward in Spring.

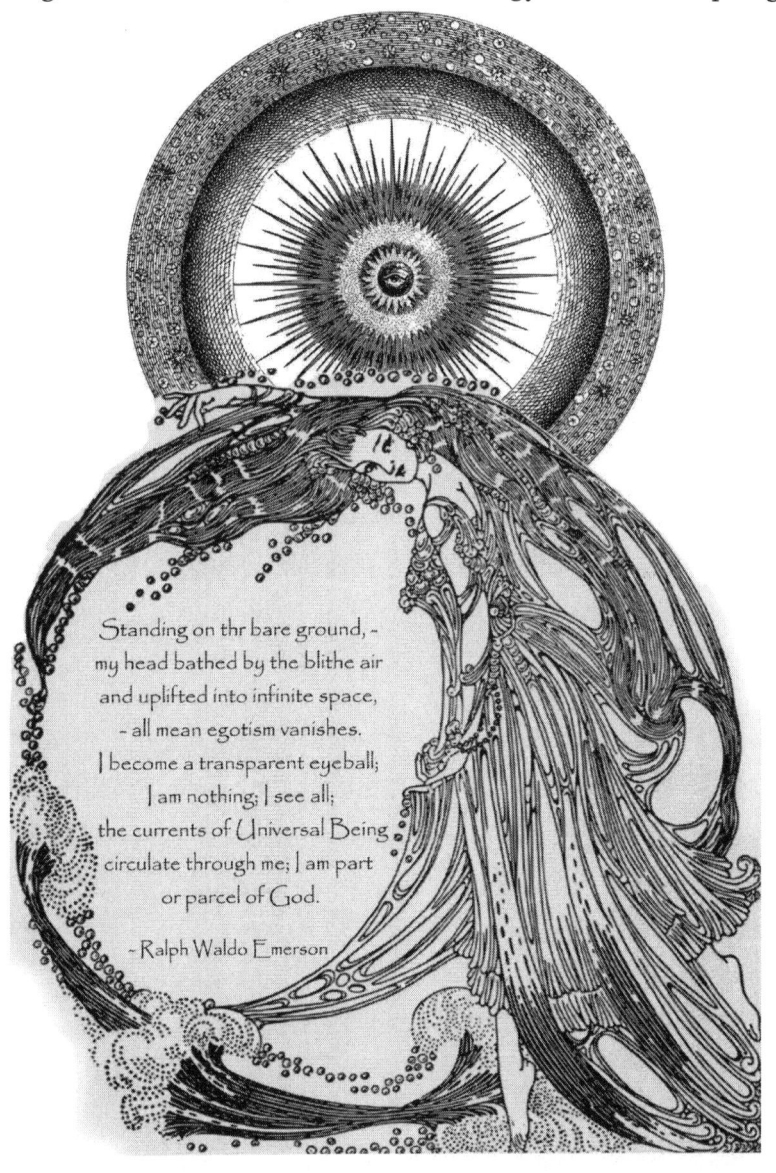

> Standing on thr bare ground, -
> my head bathed by the blithe air
> and uplifted into infinite space,
> - all mean egotism vanishes.
> I become a transparent eyeball;
> I am nothing; I see all;
> the currents of Universal Being
> circulate through me; I am part
> or parcel of God.
>
> ~ Ralph Waldo Emerson

# WHAT TO AVOID

Avoid squandering Lifeforce energy. Unhealthy eating, drinking, and lifestyle habits deplete Lifeforce energy. Constant stimulation of the senses dissipates Lifeforce energy stored in the internal organs – energy that could be conserved for maintaining health. Avoid overtaxing the body with excessive exercise, extreme physical challenges, and heavy physical labor. Taxing the mind and body chasing pleasures and material wealth uses up more energy that can be generated and wastes energy that could be used to repair and regenerate the body.

Avoid ingesting anything that devitalizes the body. Avoid eating dead flesh, highly processed foods, junk foods, fried foods, non-organic, microwaved and irradiated foods, and synthetic food substitutes. Avoid eating three meals every day. Avoid overeating. Avoid eating in a noisy, busy environment. Avoid eating every day. Practice intermittent fasting. Avoid excessive protein intake. Avoid foods that create acidity in the body. Cancers cannot flourish in an alkaline environment. Avoid/limit meat, dairy products, alcohol, refined sugars, high-fructose corn syrup, hydrogenated oils, refined carbohydrates, artifical additives, non-organic sodas, coffee, and grains, and pharmaceutical drugs. These poisons cause neuroinflammation, which destroys mental and physical health. Eat to create alkalinity, immunity, and vitality.

Avoid GMOs, factory-farmed and laboratory-manufactured animal products, fluoride, chlorine, glyphosate, phthalates, mercury, x-rays, pharmaceutical drugs, street drugs, artificial sweeteners, and toxic personal care and household cleaning products, including makeup, nail polish, nail polish remover, shampoo, conditioner, soap, hand sanitizer, artificial scents, colognes, perfumes, laundry detergents, dryer sheets, fabric softeners, and air fresheners. All these products destroy mental and physical health. Use natural, non-toxic, plant-based, organic products and medicines.

Avoid suppressing natural bodily functions, such as burping, sneezing, and farting. Be mindful and respectful of others, but don't hold your farts, don't hold your pee, and poop when you feel the need. Allowing the body to function normally, without hindrance and shame, increases personal power.

Avoid activities that devitalize the body, including wearing rubber soled shoes; staying indoors; watching TV; staring at screens; video gaming; listening to low-vibrational music; exposure to chemicals, carcinogens, and disharmonious frequencies; lying, manipulating, doing harm, and violating Natural Law; following news and politics; city living; and participating in the matrix of enslavement. Avoid toxic thoughts, speech, people, relationships, jobs, environments, and information. Stop doing what is unnecessary, unhelpful, unreasonable, dishonest, dishonorable, harmful, and destructive to self and society in order to conserve and protect energy, and to reveal the real self. When energy is conserved, there is more available for higher purposes – for the unfoldment, discipline, and growth of our higher nature.

Avoid being sedentary, sitting for hours, and interfacing with life predominantly through screens/black mirrors.

Avoid/limit technologies that create dopamine addiction, including cell phones, laptops, personal computers, video games, and 'smart' devices. From the perspective of the evolution of human consciousness, technology can be both a change agent and a hindrance. Although more information is shared more widely and quickly, these devices deter us from what we are here to do. Instead of looking inward and to Nature for inspiration, solutions, and answers, most people look to the nearest screen. Our predators created and introduced addictive screen technologies to disconnect us from our Divine nature and Nature, to capture our attention and direct our focus, hijack our creative power, maintain control, ensure our enslavement, and expedite the devolution of humankind.

Soul evolution takes place through activations of one's heart, through expansion of consciousness, through acts of loving kindness, through innerwork, energywork, sacred plant medicines, and through meditation – not through a screen. Screen technologies have been designed to stop us from being human and from being connected to Earth, to Nature, to each other, and to Divine Love. Screen technologies offer endless distractions from achieving self-mastery and being fully present – grounded, powerful, healthy, radiating Light, and embodying and emanating Love. Living life through a screen is disempowering and dehumanizing. Devices are divisive vices. The fact that most children are addicted to and relating to life through screens signals the demise of humankind. Avoid living life primarily through screens.

*"The world is not real in the way you think it is. It is a reality generation machine of some kind that can produce endless rabbit holes and show both sides of conflicting information at the same time. Collecting all the details of how everything works here is pointless. Reality investigation of endless lies, fraud, deception, and corruption is collecting evidence for what we already know is true, but refuse to accept.*

*The first goal of the psychopathic system is to recruit your participation through systems and screens. Reaching out to embrace it breathes life into it, creating a loop where it strengthens itself at the demise of the collective consciousness of the remaining souls. Its second goal is to hide you from your true self, to convince you that you are anything other than yourself, and to distract you from discovering your true self. The more one chooses to freely engage with the system and its screens, the more Divine essence evaporates out of your soulstuff, out of your light, until one essentially loses oneself to this place.*

*This place provides all that is needed to build up spiritual muscle and be free:*

*Step One: Disengage from the entire system.*

*Never take its fruit.*

*Never turn energy in its direction.*

*Step Two: Look for all answers inside yourself,*

*never from the screen or an "authority."*
**Step Three:** *When in doubt, make the human decision. Use the heart, not the head, to make decisions. Operate through feeling and abandon the logical mind.*
**Step Four:** *Ignore the lies and noise from the screen and the system about who you are and what you are capable of and discover your true self.*
**Step Five:** *Ignore the distractions, deceptions, and misinformation about how you should live your life, and develop spiritually.*
**Step Six:** *For the rest of your life always carry yourself as a massively important, immortal entity because that is what you are."*

– MATTHEW MCKINELY[93]

Avoid all vaccinations, flu shots, and all experimental injectables. Vaccines and pharmaceutical drugs are primary weapons in the parasites' arsenal. These poisons are intended to destroy our physical integrity, our innate defense system, and our ability to think clearly and independently, to reproduce, to connect with God, and enjoy life as human beings with optimal health and well-being. You are risking your life with every injection because there are ingredients that destroy empathy, intelligence, fertility, soul connection,

---

[93] FreeVoice – Lifting The Veil: https://freevoice.io/YouTube and other platforms: Quantum of Conscience. https://www.youtube.com/channel/UCA3tbHe2O7qoryWamx696fA

and the human genome,[94] Do not allow black magic into your body or your blood, or into the bodies of children via needles. Vaccinating newborns and children is unconscionable, criminal, and genocidal.[95]

> *"People listen to this closely – vaccines always have been a method of mass destruction, a method of depopulation, and a method of creating customers for life. This is truly a control weapon to make you be either chronically sick, kill you, or put you into subjugation in the transhumanism movement for the rest of your life."*
>
> – Dr Sherri Tenpenny [96]

The COVID-19 jabs are the most deadly jabs ever released. These shots are bioweapons, not vaccinations, because they do not prevent re-infection or contagion. Hundreds of thousands of recipients have died within 6 months of being "fully

---

[94] Doerfler, W. *Adenoviral Vector DNA- and SARS-CoV-2 mRNA-Based Covid-19 Vaccines: Possible Integration into the Human Genome - Are Adenoviral Genes Expressed in Vector-based Vaccines?*. Virus research. Vol. 302 (2021). https://www.ncbi.nlm.nih.gov/pmc/articles/PMC8168329/

[95] Children's Health Defense Team, *'Vaccine Secrets': What Parents Should Know Before They Vaccinate Their Kids*, 17 March 2021. https://childrenshealthdefense.org/defender/vaccine-secrets-parents-should-know-before-vaccinate/

[96] Bitchute: *Dr Sherri Tenpenny Explains How the Depopulation mRNA Vaccines Will Start Working in 3-6 Months*. Sergeant Major. 2 June 2021 https://www.bitchute.com/video/thgHE7VUsDrn/?fbclid=IwAR3NY3xSnHaZBIxU_Ufsrk7A4peKl5D8RHsmfzQP00izwp6_jc0RLVNKL5U

vaccinated" - more than 30 people per day in the US alone - but deaths are underreported and not reported as vaccine deaths.[97] All previous vaccine trials were stopped before the total death toll reached 50![98] Variants are fabricated to hide jab injuries. Despite death threats, discreditation, job loss, public ridicule, censorship, cancel culture, and censorship, doctors, scientists, and individuals with integrity, courage, wisdom, and compassion, are demanding for the immediate cessation of all CV jab programs worldwide.

*"This is serious medical science, and you're mucking around with billions of people's health for the most tenuous of reasons, and it's totally and utterly unacceptable. When it comes to injecting this stuff into the arms of children, I call that state-sanctioned child abuse of the most monstrous scale. It is utterly unacceptable, and it should stop immediately. Doctors are culpable of extreme medical malpractice. It is medical negligence of the highest order to be following government orders when you know it is doing harm. The truth will out. Heads will*

---

[97] Rumble: ATTORNEY THOMAS RENZ "We Got Them. Fact Check This!" ALL NEW WHISTLEBLOWER INFO. BookitCJ. 27 September 2021
https://rumble.com/vn12v1-attorney-thomas-renz-we-got-them.-fact-check-this-all-new-whistleblower-inf.html

[98] Schmeck, H. *Swine Flu Program is Halted in 9 States as 3 Dies After Shots.* www.nytimes.com 13 October 1976
https://www.nytimes.com/1976/10/13/archives/swine-flu-prograrm-is-halted-in-9-states-as-3-die-after-shots.html

*roll. There will be blood in the gutter, and that will happen very soon. So many are culpable here –politicians, medical colleges, regulatory bodies, media, physicians – all are of culpable of the most terrible crime committed against Humanity."*

- Dr Roger Hodkinson[99]

Natural immunity and acquired immunity are unsurpassable. Vaccinating those with immunity is medical malpractice. Multitudes are being reinfected and dying after being "fully vaccinated," which proves that the vaccines lack both efficacy and safety, and makes vaccine passports completely null and void.[100]

*"The only sure thing a vaccine 'passport' or verification proves is that somebody complied with advice or mandates. It does not guarantee that the person has any level of immunity."*

- Sharyl Attkisson [101]

---

[99] Bitchute: *Urgent Message from Dr. Roger Hodkinson Regarding the Vaccine.* TruthVideos1984. 13 June 2021.
https://www.bitchute.com/video/PKc7qogwqNjr/

[100] Huff, E. *Nearly all "covid" deaths in September occurred in the fully vaccinated* . www.naturalnews.com 10 Octerber 2021
https://www.naturalnews.com/2021-10-10-nearly-all-covid-deaths-september-fully-vaccinated.html

[101] Mercola, J, *Why Vaccine Passports Must Be Rejected.* www.articles.mercola.com 28 August 2021
https://articles.mercola.com/sites/articles/archive/2021/08/28/

> *"The vaccine passports are literally the end of human liberty in the West if the plan unfolds as planned."*
>
> – Naomi Wolf [102]

Ingredients in the shots and mechanisms of injury are being discovered as the injection experiment proceeds despite repeated warnings, desperate pleas, and heartbreaking testimonies from victims and their families. Millions are experiencing serious adverse reactions and permanent injuries immediately, and within hours, days, weeks and months of the shots, including vascular damage, blood clots, strokes, heart attacks, myocarditis, breathing difficulties, neurological damage, seizures, loss of taste, loss of smell, loss of hearing, hair loss, loss of limbs, Bell's palsy, Guillain-Barre syndrome, Multiple Sclerosis, Creutzfeldt-Jakob (prion) disease, VAIDS[103], rashes, boils, shingles and herpes simplex activations, regrowth of cancers, new cancers, excruciating pain, headaches, migraines, inability to sleep, vertigo, visual disturbances, blurred vision, blindness, impaired thinking, difficulty speaking, dementia, unshakeable brain fog and fatigue, insomnia, tics, eye twitches, paralysis,

---

vaccine-passports.aspx
https://sharylattkisson.com/

[102] Rumble: *Vaccine Passports Will Cause the Economic Collapse of America.* Bannon's War Room. 23 August 2021
https://rumble.com/vllfqg-vaccine-passports-will-cause-the-economic-collapse-of-america.html
https://drnaomiwolf.com/

[103] Vaccine Acquired Immunodeficiency Syndrome.

impotence, menstrual irregularities, vaginal ulcers, infertility, miscarriages, stillbirths, birth deformities,[104] vaccidents,[105] and soul severance.[106] Babies have died from drinking the beastmilk of their recently jabbed mothers.[107] More and new injuries are reported every day.

Most deaths and injuries are the result of the catastrophic damage caused to the human body by synthetic spike proteins, which are being manufactured in the bodies of injection recipients. Magnetofection (magnetic, force-based, gene transfer technology) in the jabs hacks innate defense and inserts artifical mRNA coding information into cells that instructs ribosomes to manufacture synthetic spike proteins – SARS-CoV-2 spike proteins – in an uncontrolled fashion.

---

[104] Vaccine Adverse Effect Reporting System: https://vaers.hhs.gov/data.html
Open VAERS: https://www.openvaers.com/index.php
Yellow Card Scheme: https://yellowcard.mhra.gov.uk/
https://www.gov.uk/government/publications/coronavirus-covid-19-vaccine-adverse-reactions/coronavirus-vaccine-summary-of-yellow-card-reporting
EurdaVigilance – European Database of suspected adverse drug reaction reports:
https://www.adrreports.eu/en/index.html
Australian Therapeutic Goods Administration:
https://www.tga.gov.au/database-adverse-event-notifications-daen

[105] Accidents while driving and flying following receipt of the shot due to sudden death or loss of consciousness and/or motor control

[106] Anonymous. Covid vaccine cuts people off spiritually-personal experience. www.human-synthesis.ghost.io 12 December 2021
https://human-synthesis.ghost.io/2021/12/12/covid-vaccine-cuts-people-off-spiritually/

[107] Li, S. *COVID-19 Report: Breastfeeding Baby Dies After Mother Receives Pfizer Vaccine.* www.visiontimes.com 30 April 2021
https://www.visiontimes.com/2021/04/30/covid-19-report-breastfeeding-baby-dies-after-mother-receives-pfizer-vaccine.html

Spike proteins circulate throughout the entire body via the blood and attach to ACE2 receptors located in all organs and tissues throughout the body, which prevents normal functioning. They break through the blood brain barrier, modify proteins in brain, cause neurological damage, damage the cardiovascular system and endothelial cells, and cause pulmonary hypertension. Spike proteins accumulate in, damage, and manipulate genes in the spleen, liver, lungs, adrenal glands, bone marrow, large intestine, uterine lining, placenta, ovaries, testes, and other organs. These spike proteins are designed to destroy reproductive ability in females by impairing egg development and placenta function and in men by immobilizing and denaturing sperm.

Spike proteins are found in secreta (urine, saliva, nasopharyngeal fluid, breathe, sweat, breast milk, sperm, vaginal fluids), excreta (feces), and skin (sores, wounds, and pustules). Minimal exposure to spike proteins can bring about long-term changes in gene expression. These spike proteins hack the software of Life and are causing deaths and life-threatening health problems now and in the future. Plausible deniability will be used to hide jab injuries that will appear years from now. Humanity is being manipulated, hacked, and controlled at the genetic level.[108]

Those who chose not to participate in the experiment are also experiencing and reporting serious effects, including

---

[108] Li, S. *COVID-19 Report: Breastfeeding Baby Dies After Mother Receives Pfizer Vaccine.* www.visiontimes.com 30 April 2021
https://www.visiontimes.com/2021/04/30/covid-19-report-breastfeeding-baby-dies-after-mother-receives-pfizer-vaccine.html

migraines, rashes, breathing difficulties, heart palpitations, abnormal bleeding, nose bleeds, bruising, menstrual irregularities, miscarriages, and stillbirths as a result of the transmission of spike proteins being manufactured by jab recipients. Protection from bioweaponry is essential.[109]

***ALAWYS remember that there is NO bioweapon that can destroy or defeat a fearless, courageous, empowered, integrous, sovereign human being.***

More harmful ingredients are being discovered in the shots. Aborted fetal cells, heavy metals, glyphosate, parasites,[110] Luciferase,[111] graphene oxide,[112] and self-aware, self-assemblying, self-replicating nanoparticles have been identified. Nanotechnologies are one of the most dangerous weapons being used against us. They are invisible, insidious, in everything, and intended to control us from the inside.

---

[109] Bitchute: *Protection From Bioweaponry*. Feeling Better Naturally. 29 July 2021 https://www.bitchute.com/video/1H00r1ex69hq/. See 'Protocols' in **Resources** and **Book 2** in this series.

[110] Rumble: *Stew Peters Show. Jab: Scientist Discovers Hatching Eggs, Parasites Birthed After Injection*. 15 October 2021
https://rumble.com/vnslor-jab-scientist-discovers-hatching-eggs-parasites-birthed-after-injection.html

[111] Lindsay, R. *Luciferase Chain Reaction to ID2020*. www.natureofhealing.org 22 July 2020
https://www.natureofhealing.org/luciferase-id2020-system/

[112] Young, R. *Scanning & Transmission Electron Microscopy Reveals Graphene Oxide in CoV-19 Vaccines*. /www.drrobertyoung.com 1 October 2021
https://www.drrobertyoung.com/post/
transmission-electron-microscopy-reveals-graphene-oxide-in-cov-19-vaccines

There are nanotechnologies in vaccines, foods, drinks, cosmetics, personal care products, cleaning products, clothing, chemtrails, and PCR tests.[113]

Avoid getting tested for CV-19. PCR (Polymerase chain reaction) tests are not fit for purpose according to Kary Mullis, the inventor, before he died under mysterious (and convenient) circumstances in August 2019.[114] Tests cycles are overamplified to consistently produce false positive results, which are used to create and inflate case numbers, maintain the plandemic psyop, drive cycles of fear and panic, control populations, and remove freedom and human rights. PCR tests are contaminated with nefarious ingredients, including Ethylene oxide - a sterilizing agent, a pesticide, and a known carcinogen and hormone disruptor.[115] Nantechnologies intended to sicken, track, and control recipients have been found in the nasophayngeal COVID swabs. When inserted through the nasal passage beyond the blood brain barrier, nanobots create a cascade of calamities, including damage to cardiovascular, respiratory, nervous, and reproductive

---

[113] https://www.rivm.nl/en/nanotechnology/consumer-products
Koenig, P. *Stop COVID Testing Immediately: PCR and Quick Test Swabs May be Cancer-Causing.* www.truthunmuted.org. 30 March 2021

https://truthunmuted.org/stop-covid-testing-immediately-pcr-and-quick-test-swabs-may-be-cancer-causing/

[114] Odysee: *Kary Mullis Full Interview.* TRUTH@BalkanTruth. 10 June 2021
https://odysee.com/@BalkanTruth:1/
Kary-Mullis---The-full-interview-by-Gary-Null_HD:c?&sunset=lbrytv

[115] Ethylene Oxide Sterilization – a cancer causing agent according to the National Cancer Institute: www.cancer.gov
https://www.cancer.gov/about-cancer/causes-prevention/risk/substances/ethylene-oxide

systems.[116]

Nanotechnologies have been designed to lobotomize and sterilize humans and to prevent connection to All That Is. They are designed to spy on, monitor, control, program, and enslave us. Once inside the body, these nanotechnologies self assemble into a network that connects the body to AI (Alien Intelligence), the Internet of Bodies, an AI powered social credit system, and allows remote control of individuals via 5G to advance the transhuman agenda.[117] They will monitor internal and external activities, including biometrics, emotional responses, and physical activities, which will destroy privacy and bodily autonomy. Every move will be tracked and traced. These nanotechnologies will generate hivemind and obliterate individuality and freedom. Avoid allowing any AI and tracking technologies to enter into the body – through vaccinations, foods, beverages, clothing, medical procedures, implants, cranial implants, microchips, radio frequency chips, electronic/digital tattoos, quantum tattoos, and all brain-computer and mind-machine interfacing technologies and devices that can be put in or on the human body to control how people think, feel, and behave. Our predators intend to make it impossible for humans to participate in their beastly

---

[116] Red Voice Media. *The Stew Peters Show. COVID Nasal Swabs Examined by Scientists Reveal DANGER.* 18 October 2021
https://www.redvoicemedia.com/2021/10/covid-nasal-swabs-examined-by-scientists-reveal-danger/

[117] Rumble: *Dr. Carrie Madej: First U.S. Lab Examines "Vaccine" Vials, HORRIFIC Findings Revealed.* Stew Peters Show. 29 September 2021.
https://rumble.com/vn482j-dr.-carrie-madej-first-u.s.-lab-examines-vaccine-vials-horrific-findings-re.html

system without being microchipped and marked. Research and follow nanobot removal protocols.

> *"It also forced all people, great and small, rich and poor, free and slave, to receive a mark on their right hands or on their foreheads, so that they could not buy or sell unless they had the mark, which is the name of the beast or the number of its name. This calls for wisdom. Let the person who has insight calculate the number of the beast, for it is the number of a man. That number is 666."*
> — REVELATION 13: 16-18

Never enter a Faustian Bargain.[118]
Escape the Beast system.

> *"Nature has put into every cell the secret of its own salvation. It has put into the individual every faculty and power necessary for humans to achieve liberation from the delusions and illusions of earthly life."*
> — MANLY P. HALL[119]

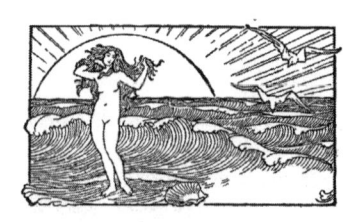

---

[118] Faust, in the legend, traded his soul to the devil in exchange for knowledge. To 'strike a Faustian bargain' is to be willing to sacrifice anything to satisfy a limitless desire for knowledge and/or power. www.dictionary.com

[119] YouTube: *How To Find Your True Purpose – Manly P. Hall – Alchemy*

# OPTIMIZING FINANCIAL POWER

It is essential to hold oneself as a sacred, seamless vessel, and in order to receive infinite abundance, there must be no cracks or leaks. One must live in integrity and in service to the greatest good. Avoid wasting money, energy, time, resources, attention, food, and other people's time, energy, attention, and resources. Express gratitude and appreciation for all resources, all manifestations, and all opportunities to make a difference in the world.

The secret to abundance is to share what one has (energy, time, money, food, shelter, material objects) and what one knows to be true with others. When we share higher knowledge, wisdom, and Truth with others, there is no limit to the abundance that we receive – more information, deeper understanding, insights, improved health, harmonious relationships, practices, siddhis[120], and Grace. To receive greater abundance, increase what you give to others and find a truth and share it, even if it challenges existing beliefs and public opinion and you feel uncomfortable or terrified.

---

– *Metaphysics – Philosophy.* MindPodNetwork, 2 October 2019. https://www.youtube.com/watch?v=EGhrhe1YAn4

Adams, M. IT'S REAL: Science paper documents *"self-assembled magnetic nanosystems" for cybernetic biocircuitry interface and control systems in humans, including "DNA hydrogel" tech.* www.naturalnews.com 20 July 2021 https://www.naturalnews.com/2021-07-20-science-paper-documents-self-assembled-magnetic-nanosystems-for-cybernetic-biocircuitry-interface.html

[120] Siddhis are supernatural and paranormal powers, abilities, and skills that can arise spontaneously or be developed over time by intense spiritual practices. Examples include psychic powers, levitation, bilocation, and access to the Akashic Records (the eternal records of all souls).

Becoming vulnerable in this way makes one invulnerable.

Practice right livelihood. Engaging in work that is fulfilling, enjoyable, in alignment with the principles of Natural Law, and serving the highest good of all increases Life Force energy and personal power, improves physical and mental health, and contributes to the freedom and future of Humanity. Engaging in work, or any activity, without love and gratitude depletes Lifeforce energy.

**Love what you do to increase LifeForce energy.**

Invest in oneself so one can better serve God. Invest in improving your health, value, and competence. Invest in quality, organic food, and supplements. Invest in purifying water. Invest in healing, detoxifying, self-improvement, and expansion of consciousness. Invest in bodywork. Invest in growing food, planting trees and fruit trees, and restoring and beautifying Earth. Invest in sustainable energy, sustainable food production, healing technologies, environmental restoration, and rewilding of self and Earth. Invest in a clean, safe, peaceful, equitable, abundant world for all.

Make a budget and stick to it. Pay bills on time with gratitude. Avoid debt. Give more than you receive. Share your time, energy, attention, resources, skills, and gifts generously. Remove mental blocks to abundance and learn to receive. Tip generously.

Help others to help themselves. Support those who are doing the Great Work.[121]

Bank Karma. Do good deeds. Make someone else's day/life

---

[121] The rescue of a soul from the forces that bind it.

better. Practice random acts of kindness and charity. Make someone else's life better. Feed people.

> *"If you cultivate good will and a sincere desire to help others in every transaction, it will be one of the best investments you have ever made."*
> – WALLACE D. WATTLES[122]

Withdraw financial support from all systems of enslavement. Establish and use alternative economies and energy exchange systems.

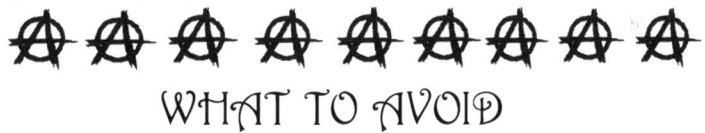

## WHAT TO AVOID

Avoid making money more important than people and the planet. Avoid greed for money, material possesions, food, fame, excitement, and physical pleasures. Greed can never be satiated. The more you obtain, the more you will crave, and the more you crave, the more you will scheme to satisfy those cravings, which depletes Lifeforce energy. Address addictions. Avoid hoarding and wasting money. Buy only what is essential. Stop buying plastics and single use products, and stop creating waste. Avoid being a wage slave. Avoid investing in genocide and ecocide.

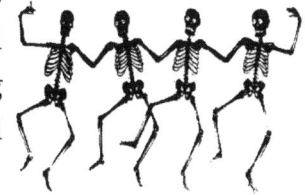

---

[122] YouTube: *Personal Power Course, Wallace D Wattles.* Giving Voice to the Wisdom of the Ages. 4 March 2021.
https://www.youtube.com/watch?v=t8B07vpASBI&t=6769s.

# INCREASING PERSONAL POWER

*"For where two or three are gathered together in my name, there am I in the midst of them."*
- Matthew 18:20 (KJV)

When we come together physically, we are empowered by the merging and synergizing of the fields of energy that radiate from every loving heart. Standing more than two meters (six feet) apart (a "public health" regulation imposed during the scamdemic) is completely disempowering, because our all-powerful fields of Love/heart energy are not synchronous. Social/physical distancing has been enforced to weaken us energetically, individually and collectively. Being physically together with other open-hearted human beings is one of the most empowering things we can do. The force of Love is amplified exponentially, and New Earth and the Fifth Dimension is tangible.

Humans need loving touch to thrive. Making human connections with other people is empowering. Hug. Smile. Make eye contact. Listen. Share. Help. In a safe situation, offer and receive loving, non-sexual touch. A hand massage. A foot massage. A back massage. Make love if that is an option. Harnessing sexual energy to serve the common good is a highly effective way to increase personal power. Dedicating and offering the energy of love-making and self-pleasuring to the highest good of all is an empowering practice that changes reality.

***"Too often we underestimate the power of a touch, a smile, a kind word, a listening ear, an honest compliment, or the smallest act of caring, all of which have the potential to turn a life around."***
– Leo F. Buscaglia

Seek opportunities to be with others – to share a meal, to pray, meditate, sing, dance, play, express gratitude, talk story, make music, make art, share wisdom, watch a sunrise/sunset, grow food, picnic in a park, march for freedom, and enjoy and celebrate Life. Strive to become more likeable, more charismatic, more trustworthy, more helpful, more kindhearted, and more community minded. Start locally. Find your tribe. Create a soul family. Build Resilience circles.[123] We are an interdependent species, and strengthening social connections strengthens personal power.

Everything is interconnected and interdependent. We are all connected. Cultivate kinship with all relations. Take every opportunity to connect with all life forms – animals, birds, trees, plants, nature spirits, celestial bodies, and other unseen, benevolent intelligences. Build and maintain right relationships with human and animal neighbors. Be a friend to make a friend. Be a good parent, a good partner, a mentor, a student, a beacon of Light. Fulfill the responsibilities and duties of these roles to the best of your ability. Demonstrate affection and appreciation. Say "I love you" and "thank you."

---

[123] Small groups of 10-20 people who come together to increase personal security during challenging times. www.localcircles.org

Be an active member of a group that is focused on creating peace, Love, New Earth, and the highest good for all.

***Take care of Nature,
and Nature will take care of you.***

# WHAT TO AVOID

Avoide the Metaverse. Avoid staying behind a screen. Staying still. Staying indoors. Staying at home. Staying fearful. Stagnating. Staying small. Staying enslaved. Living a lie. Feeding the parasites with negative emotions. Participating in the old paradigm.

# OPTIMIZING PERSONAL POWER

Doing just one of the practices that promote spiritual power, mind power, will power, sexual power, financial power, and/or community power once will increase personal power. Doing more than one for weeks, months, and years is most empowering. Many practices and methods for increasing personal power can be safely combined to increase the effects. For example: barefoot running on the beach; sungazing barefoot while standing on wet grass; meditating in Nature and near an altar; and making Love on the Earth.

***Feel your power intensifying
every day.***

# CO-CREATING NEW EARTH

We are the Creators. We are the ones with all the power. We have the juice, the good stuff, and the soulstuff. We have what low vibrational, parasitic lifeforms want above all else. Our predators have no true power and no way to manifest anything without compliant human beings, because they have no creative abilities, no originality, no Love, and no Light – which is why they hijack the Divine creative power of human beings to manifest their satanic world – a world of evil, greed, deception, inversion, perversion, and vampirism. Without our energy, attention, consent, and participation, they are powerless, and their systems of enslavement will collapse. It is time to withdraw all energy, attention, consent, and participation. It is time to claim our Divine power and use it to establish a reality based in Love, Truth, and Freedom.

Each of us needs to be as powerful as possible because it is the combined energy of Love in our hearts that is destroying the fear-based, false reality matrix and co-creating the love-based reality of New Earth. Not only do we need to co-create a beautiful, new Earth by feeling and radiating Love, peace, and joy as fully as possible as often as possible, but we also need to defend ourselves from escalating attacks upon our physical, mental, spiritual, and social health. Increasing personal power is an essential daily practice, as the war on consciousness has escalated. Systems of control and torture are tightening in order to extract as much low vibrational energy (fear, anxiety, confusion, desperation, frustration, irritability, impatience, anger, rage, pain, and panic) from humankind as possible before their imminent collapse, demise, and disappearance. The parasites know their time is up, and they are taking adavatge of their last opportunity to gorge themselves on low vibrational energy.

For Humanity to transcend from a fear-based reality to a loved-based reality, each of us needs to be fully empowered, because it is our collective power, shared visioning, and courageous actions that will bring New Earth into physicality. Each of us is a key to the re-establishment and unfolding of our organic timeline and the co-creation of the New Earth through evolution of consciousness, co-operation, and collaboration. The best contribution one can make to this extraordinary transfiguration of our species is to embody the greatest Love, Light, peace, joy, and wisdom as possible. And to be self-aware, grounded, balanced, vigilant, and living in alignment with Truth, with God, with Love, with Higher Self, ancestors, guides, Nature, and with Natural Law. We need to be resilient, courageous, disciplined, ungovernable, invincible, and prepared to fight and die for our freedom.

**The real revolution is the evolution of consciousness.**

It is most beneficial to use personal power to raise one's vibrational frequency[124]; broaden perception; radiate peace,

---

[124] YouTube: *20 Easy ways to Raise Your Vibration: Essential Information for all Human Beings*. Feeling Better Naturally, 18 December 2020. https://www.youtube.com/watch?v=H9yKlvevu1c

love, and joy; share wisdom; create art, music, and beauty; grow and share food; help others; relax, enjoy life, and allow Divine Love to flow. Using personal power to expand consciousness is the best investment in the future.

Using personal power to protect those who are weak, vulnerable, and suffering, particularly elders and children, is imperative. Those who talk about children being the hope for the future are seriously deluded. It is the children who are being targeted, poisoned, and tortured from before birth to prevent their natural unfoldment. Children are not resilient. Children are easily traumatized for life. Most children are being by raised/damaged by parents who are suffering from multigenerational trauma. Most parents repeat cycles of abuse. Most children are living in domestic hell, in war zones, in fear, in uncertainty, in emotional. intellectual, material, and spiritual poverty, in front of screens designed to disconnect, lobotomize, and dehumanize. They are being brainwashed, sexualized, politicized, and zombified by public education, TV, Disney, movies, video games, and online schooling, learning, gaming, and socializing; poisoned by "foods," sugar, and "medications;" brain-damaged, DNA-damaged, immune-compromised, and sterilized by vaccines; and permanently psychologically scarred and brain damaged by mask wearing, social/physical distancing, sustained narratives of terror, and enforced deprivation from oxygen, friends, community, sunlight, outdoor play, and Nature. Nearly every child on Earth is being subjected to several forms of serious torture that is causing irreparable damage to that child's physical, psychological, emotional, spiritual, and social health. The damage being done to children by their own parents, schools, and "medical staff" is pure evil and ensures that most children will never reach their full potential.

We transgress Humanity when we do not care for, protect, nurture, or educate our children about right ways of living. Until parents, politicians, teachers, doctors, and other ignorant, uncaring adults stop abusing and poisoning children, children will become adults who do not know how to be human and do not have a connection to other people, God, or Nature. Those who care about the future of our children and our species need to take immediate action to protect children from further wickedness, and to ensure they learn how to be human, how to be responsible and take care of themselves and their home, how to give and receive love, and how to live in harmony with others and with Nature as a matter of the greatest urgency.

Two of the greatest blessings of this virus event are the increase in homebirths, which prevents the life-long imprint of fear upon newborns, and the rise in homeschooling, which prevents government-approved brainwashing and publicly sanctioned child torture. Children are not being educated in public schools. Their minds and their lives are being destroyed. They are being programmed to be fearful, ignorant, narcissistic, cowardly, passive, sick debt slaves. All abuse of children must end immediately or Humanity will end.

Despite the insanity of current events, there is every reason for faith and optimism. Thanks to the evil genius of

Q,[125] there are now millions more humans who understand and abhor the satanic "Agenda 2030," and who are prepared to make personal sacrifices and die for freedom. Those of us who know the truth about what is happening on Earth are the majority, and we are not alone. Our Cosmic family of Light is all-powerful and present for our transfiguration, and we have God/good on our side. There are countless beings playing roles that serve both our evolution and theirs, all according to Divine Will. Our galactic family is with us at this time of human quickening, to support us as we break free, alchemize our souls, embody the luminescence of our quintessence, and come together to co-create New Earth.

> *"We are many. They are few."*
> *Just say, "No," and it's all over."*
> — David Icke[126]

Freedom is ours. Power is ours. The future is ours. The vibrational frequency of Earth has increased evidenced by the Schumann Resonances, the heartbeat of Earth, which is literally off the charts. Earth is being flooded with photonic light activating the New Earth timeline and template, DNA

---

[125] Q is a psyop that exposes the truth about the enslavement of Humanity in a satanic blood cult while pretending to be an insurgency that will free us and hold those who have perpetrated crimes against Humanity accountable for their evil deeds. Q uses Savior programming to keep believers passive, hiding behind a keyboard, unconsciously serving evil, and ineffective in changing anything.

[126] YouTube: *What's Next For Maxwell*. Shaun Attwood. 28 August 2020. https://www.youtube.com/watch?v=ec7NBKMlINk&feature=youtu.be

codes, ancient memories, high frequency potentialities, and inherent, superluminal Divinity. The planets are aligned with energy signatures for deconstruction of the old paradigm, purging, cleansing, clearing, transformation, ascension, and freedom. All that has a lower frequency (all systems, structures, societies, and beings with low vibrational energy- greed, selfishness, hatred, fear, control, deceipt, and evil) can no longer be sustained and are being dismantled, dissolved, and expelled. All masks are coming off in preparation for the externalization of the Hierarchy.

The vibratory frequency of Earth is now the frequency of Divine Love, and all that has a lower frequency is on its way out of existence – but not without chaos and resistance, which is why we need to be fully empowered. It is essential to understand that under the command of Love, a new Cosmic cycle is upon us - the Age of Aquarius, the Satya Yuga, the Golden Age, Pacha Kuti (the over turning), New Earth. The apocalypse is here, the collapse of the old, fear-based paradigm is well underway, and the creation of a new, love-based paradigm has taken root. Divine Love is anchored and afire in the hearts of millions of humans and all benevolent beings throughout the Cosmos. Love is the most powerful force on Earth, and Love now holds dominion. New Earth is here any time one chooses to embrace it.

**We co-create New Earth every time we choose to feel, express, share, create, and make Love.**

It is essential to understand that the parasites are

distracting us from embodying Love and living in New Earth through screen technologies that broadcast their evil clown shows, diabolical theatrics, psyops, false flags, "news," and other attention grabbers. Screens are constantly pumping out lies, half-truths, disinformation, and fearporn, perpetuating and enforcing a sinister agenda. When we stop paying attention to, and giving energy to, the antics of the evil ones, stop being distracted, transfixed, and ruled by screens, and stop participating in and complying with their systems of control, we can feel, experience, and embody infinitely more Love/Light. The parasites' most effective strategy has been to distract humans from receiving Love/Light. As more people realize how they are being deceived, controlled, and played, and choose not to comply, and to reconnect with Nature/Earth/God, embody Divine Love and power and take right action, the Great Reset will remain a globalist's wet dream.

### *Now is the time for mass non-compliance.*

From the highest perspective, only Love is real, there is no evil, and there are no "bad guys." There is Natural Law and there are consequences for all thoughts, words, and actions. A soul chooses a life in this paradoxical, earthly realm of duality where there is good and evil for the opportunity to evolve like nowhere else in the Cosmos. Soul evolution is the reason for embodiment. There are no exceptions and no victims. There are endless opportunities for spiritual growth and evolution.

What we see out in the world is a reflection of what lies within – the good, the bad, and the ugly. All that is good that manifests in the world is the outpicturing of Divine Love within every human being. All that is evil that manifests on Earth is the outpicturing of unexamined darkness within every human being. All that unfolds on the world stage is in accordance with God's Will – the Divine Plan for the highest good of all – and serves to catalyze the evolutionary journey of Earth and all Her inhabitants from fear to Love.

What we are witnessing and experiencing are the events conditions, and initiatory forces necessary to transform Humanity from a fear-driven species to a species driven by Love, our natural state. Behold the glorious presence of New Earth as more evidence appears daily and give thanks. Behold the pathetic death throes of the evil empire and give thanks for their end days. The predator class is serving Divine Will, the highest good for all, and playing the role we asked and need them to play in order to propel us out of enslavement and onto our organic timeline. All that is transpiring is to awaken humankind from a deep coma to the reality of tyranny, to stimulate the free will of the masses, to catapult human beings out of ignorance and complacency into action, to claim sovereignty, accept full responsibility, unite, and co-create the reality that is our inalienable birthright. Prayers for freedom are being answered. The skullduggery and the shitshow that we are witnessing are what is needed to break the dreamspell and free humankind from the shackles of fear and delusion, the illusions of separation and time,[127]

---

[127] All suffering, destruction, entropy, and death is connected to the illusion of time.

and the cancerous tyranny of evil. It is empowering to be grateful for opportunities for unification, spiritual growth, sovereignty, and evolution that are present and forgive the evildoers for the evil deeds that they perpetrate. These loveless, soulless entities are serving the highest good of all, even though it may not look or feel that way. Know that there are consequences for all violations of Natural Law and that Love has already won, regardless of what is taking place worldwide. All outward manifestations of fear and chaos are temporary illusions. Nothing will stop what is coming.

We are all on this spiraling, cyclical, hero's journey undergoing metamorphosis together, and celestial bodies are aligned to empower the awakening and transfiguration of humankind and Earth. Global uprising against totalitarianism is mounting, as the planets line up to usher in the dawn of an Aquarian age. New Earth is already here, and the future is fluid and ours to shape with every thought word, and action. Through self-sacrifice, self-actualization, unity consciousness, systemic co-operation, and Grace, we will put ALL our differences aside – gender, race, religion, politics, class, generation, medical status – and unite against our common enemy. We will stand together as One in Unity consciousness, indivisible and invincible, and expand the unified forcefield of Love and anchor the Divine Blueprint to ensure the glorious future of Humanity in the Age of Light. One People – One Planet. This is the only way Humanity will survive and thrive. And thrive we will!

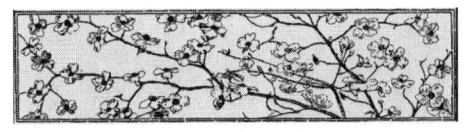

> *"It is in crisis where the greatest breakthroughs are possible. Within these tension points in human history lies the seed of what becomes the future."*
> – WILLIAM MEADER[128]

It is time to celebrate the end of the Great Darkness and rejoice! The Sacred Tribe is gathering on Earth and throughout the Cosmos, and we are countless. Wave upon wave of Divine Light is cleansing Earth of evil, dispelling black magic, dissolving the boundaries of rigid dogmas, superstition, separation, and fear, and activating unity consciousness. It is time to shine effulgently in this Age of Light, of Truth, equality, and equanimity. Of Spiritual Singularity.[129] Through evermore wondrous, heart-centered, nature-based, multi-dimensional, egalitarian living, we actualize New Earth and seed a future in which we co-create, procreate, communicate, heal, interact, transact, keep the peace, teach our children, and feed ourselves, and all our relations with Love, for the highest good of all.

> *"The secret of changes is to focus all your energy, not on fighting the old, but on building the new."*
> – SOCRATES

We are the grassroots. the groundswell, the tsunami,

---

[128] www.meader.org

[129] YouTube: Vanessa VA https://www.youtube.com/channel/UChNMIAVEeqHUrDAvtxBqgOA (Also on other platforms.)

and the tidal wave of change. We are fierce warriors for freedom. We are lucid dreamers, Divine doulas, alchemical midwives, and architects of the future. We are modern mystics, metaphysicians, and magicians. We are becoming *Homo luminous, Homo spiritualis,* and *Homo celestus.* We are the ones we have been waiting for, and it is time to claim our genetic heritage, our Divine heritage, and our galactic heritage. It is a great honor for any soul to be here now to birth New Earth. It is our responsibility to do so with the fullness of our being, so that we manifest the brightest, most beauteous, and abundant world with the highest octaves of Love/Light.

*"We stand at the threshold of a great dawning.*
*Something deep within Life is changing,*
*an era is ending, and at the very core of creation,*
*something new is being born.*
*We are awakening from a long and collective sleep.*
*An invitro dream deep within the womb*
*of our mother Gaia.*
*We are awakening.*
*A planetary birthing,*
*emerging from the amniotic fluid.*
*A new species.*
*A new Man/Woman of the stars.*
*Birthing into a family of Light.*
*Leaving behind old paradigms and outdated*
*modalities, and embracing ourselves*
*as part of the Whole, fractal expressions*
*of a unified field of consciousness.*

*Walk with an open heart, and recognize
something so vast on this planet,
in this solar system, in this galaxy,
inside this universe.
Countless universes and systems of worlds
and other dimensions, intercepting and
interpenetrating in a joyous experience
of this present moment!
All things are possible!
Dare to dream, make your dreams come true,
and let yourself fly.
Be whole. Be conscious. Be free and let go.
Let life live you.
Let life be the dancer.
Simply become the dance.
The cycle of being separate is closing.
A great step in our evolution.
Into multidimensional awareness.
A new Man/Woman is being born.
Homo-Celestus.
One who can live in peace on the earth.
One who is capable of moving through
many worlds and dimensions.
One who seeks to share energy,
creativity in harmony in the spirit of co-operation.
One who can transmit peace to other worlds
and other planes of existence."*

— ANANDI SUNDANCER[130]

---

[130] http://www.anandisundancer.com/journeys-peak/

Envision our future.

How does New Earth look, feel, smell, taste, and sound to you?

Hold your vision and energize it at every opportunity..

**_Let's make the birth of New Earth orgasmic!_**

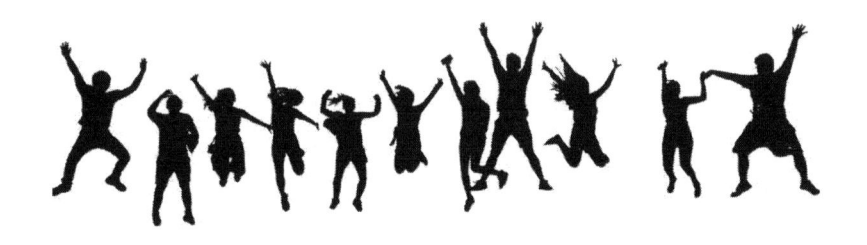

May the sun bring you
new energy by day.

May the moon softly restore
you by night.

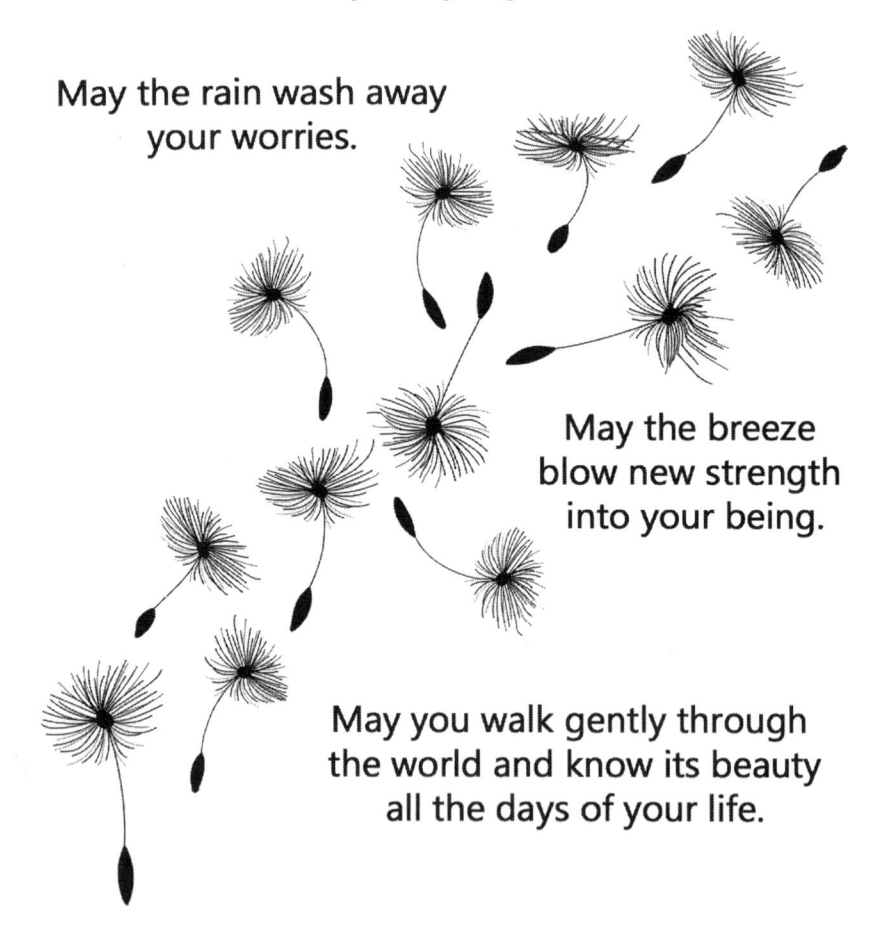

May the rain wash away
your worries.

May the breeze
blow new strength
into your being.

May you walk gently through
the world and know its beauty
all the days of your life.

APACHE BLESSING

# A VISION FOR NEW EARTH: TERRA NOVA

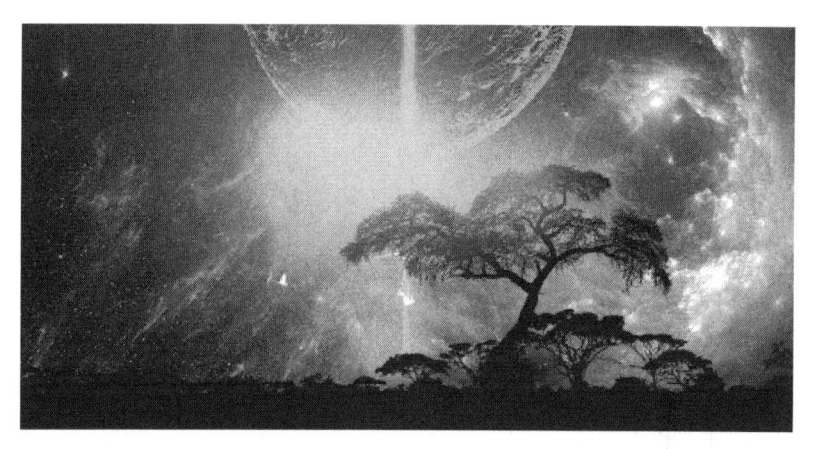

> *"What most don't realize is that New Earth is seeded. It's here, primed, ready, willing, and waiting for its Creators to awaken to create their New Earth."*
>
> – ALEX MARCOUX[131]

New Earth is cleansed, rejuvenated, rebalanced, and restored to Her pristine, resplendent form as the glistening, blue, crowning jewel of the Cosmos. New Earth is exquisite, glorious, peaceful, and bountiful. She is a living library bathed in the highest frequencies of shimmering, golden Light that optimize all life and promote soul evolution, well-being, health, and harmony. The air is clean, sweet, oxygen-rich, and invigorating. Oceans, rivers, lakes, and all bodies of waters

---

[131] Marcoux, A. *New Earth and Spiritual Ascension to the Fifth Dimension.* www.alexmarcoux.com
https://alexmarcoux.com/5d/what-is-the-new-earth-spiritual-ascension/

are purified, shining, and teeming with life. There are new and ancient species of plants and wildlife inhabiting Earth. Vast, verdant forests full of wildlife and myriad orchards of fruit trees grow abundantly. Food gardens, medical plant gardens, flower gardens, and community gardens flourish. All planetary energy centers are fully activated – chakras, ley lines, vortexes, interdimensional portals, star gates, sacred sites, megaliths, mountains, crystals, rocks, and trees. Secrets have been unlocked from Earth, and sacred places and long buried, ancient sites are revealed and activated.

Higher consciousness has birthed, and Earth is inhabited by a new species of human. Humans have shifted from separation and duality to unity consciousness and Oneness. Humans are Divinicus,[132] Homoluminous,[133] multidimensional, heart-centered, spiritually enlightened beings who love, respect, honor, cherish, and nourish Earth as the Divine being that She is. Humans are living in alignment with Natural Law, and in harmony with Earth, each other, and all beings of Love and Light throughout the Cosmos. In New Earth, there is no evil, no war, no homelessness, no poverty, no starvation, no scarcity, no corruption, no pollution, no religions, no divisions, no masters, and no slaves. The Law of the Tribe prevails – no one has more than another and no one has less than another. There is anarchy, unity, equality, peace, beauty, and infinite, unconditional love.

---

[132] https://wakeup-world.com/2013/01/28/homo-divinicus-the-shape-of-things-to-come/

[133] https://thefourwinds.com/blog/shamanism/homo-luminous-new-human/

The ancient blueprint for living is reestablished. Everything is unified by holism, wholeness, and holiness. All humans uphold the principle of Love and experience Oneness with All That Is. All know the truth of existence and live in service to Prime Creator and the highest good for all. Free will is aligned with Divine Will. Individual worth comes from inside, through spiritual growth and development, evolution of consciousness, creativity, and what can be contributed to the greater good. All maintain an internal motivation of "Service to Others," rather than "Service to Self." Masculine and feminine principles within human nature are balanced and unified with Higher Self, Nature, and Source.

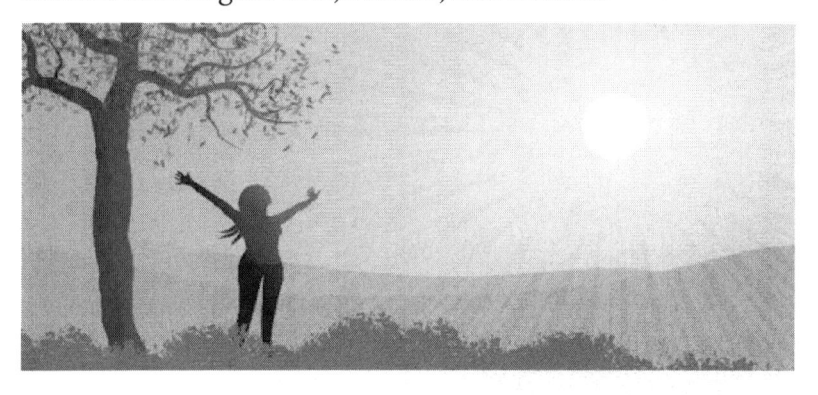

In New Earth, the world is full of light and life. Every bit of air is a carrier of truth and wisdom. Of mysteries and marvels. Of potency and potentials. Humans awaken with the sun each day to co-create a bright, new day with every elevated holy breath and a bright, new way forward in a reality anchored in Natural Law and based in Love, Truth, and Freedom. Free from life as a debt slave, humans are now able to unfurl their Divine blueprint, explore their limitless nature, fulfill their God-given potential, and enjoy life as an embodiment of Divine Love. All exercise the right to freedom of speech, freedom of movement, freedom of association and assembly, the right to body autonomy, and the right to work and retain the fruits of one's labor. Humans are free to devote themselves to soul growth, deepening in communion with Infinite Intelligence, and community building. They have time to nurture and develop relationships with seen and unseen beings throughout the Cosmos, making Earth an intergalactic civilization. All are free to be inventive and innovative, and to fulfill their full creative potential. Creativity is the driving force, reciprocity is currency, and intuition and inspiration are guides.

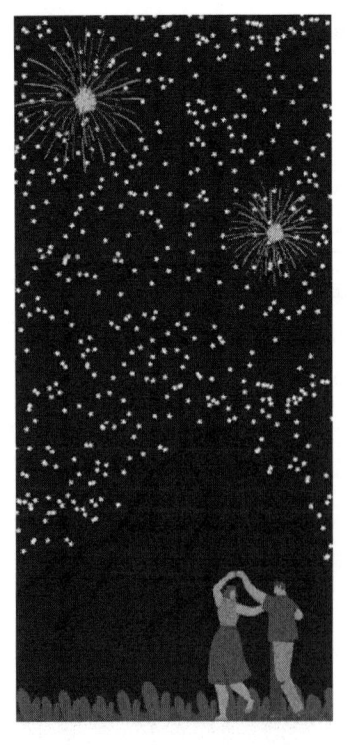

Technology serves Humanity. Humans thrive on heart-based, nature-based living. Humans enjoy omnipresent awareness and deep connections with other people, Earth-based life forms, and beings from other dimensions. All exist harmoniously, cooperatively, and joyously. There is a profound sense of belonging. Everything about everyone who exists is not only accepted, but admired, respected, recognized, and celebrated. There is a co-operative, co-passion for being that permeates life. Life is effortless, blissful, and joy-filled.

Communication is predominantly telepathic, with respect to privacy being adhered to by all. Honesty is always practiced because lying is instantly detected. Humans can access multivector consciousness and integrate information and lifetimes from other dimensions, realities, and timelines. Life is held sacred, and there are ceremonies, rituals, dances, sacred music, and group prayer and meditations. Laughter, music, movement, art, and enjoyment are daily practices. There is an abundance of leisure time. Rest, relaxation, and recreation are intentionally practiced. More time is spent in play and playing with consciousness and energy. Consciousness can do anything technology can do and more. Manifestation and terraforming are easy, and life is full of creating and expanding beauty and love.

Humans love and respect their physical reality and their physicality. Each person benefits from the physicality of Life and births well-being and upliftment for oneself. The physical body is honored as a sacred temple and treated and enjoyed accordingly. Maintaining a high vibrational frequency is natural. Physical bodies are less dense, more light-filled, and crystalline-based, rather than carbon-based, which requires less maintenance. All 12 DNA codes are fully activated by higher frequencies, making individual and collective potential limitless. Given that 93% of the function of DNA is light and sound reception and transmission, physical bodies become more refined and more ethereal, and consciousness continues to expand.

There is no longer the heavy gravitational pull of Earth, and humans have the ability to transport themselves physically above the ground, from one place to another, by the power of thought alone. Teleportation and bilocation are possible. The need for sleep and food has lessened. Most humans desire to eat simply and for pleasure. There are new and ancient varieties of highly nutritious fruits, vegetables, foods, and beverages that optimize health. Nourishment can also be drawn from the etheric body, Nature, the Sun, the Ether, and all sources of Light and Love. Motion is more fluid and graceful, and strength can be superhuman. Sexual energy is sacred and used for procreation and creation of all that serves the highest good.

Alongside humans, there are other loving, highly evolved, interdimensional beings enjoying and enhancing life on Earth. All have the awareness of the oneness of All and the allness of One. The golden rule of do unto others as one would only have done to oneself is followed at all times. All beings co-exist harmoniously and in service to Gaia, Prime Creator, and to the greatest good of all. All beings treat each other with respect, compassion, and lovingkindness. Mutually beneficial relationships between all beings are developed and nurtured. There is abundance and prosperity for all to enjoy.

In New Earth, cultural heritage is preserved, and any differences contribute to and integrate into the whole. All differences blend like fragrances in a flower garden where all the different flowers contribute their bouquet to the overall perfume. Each individual flower remains distinct with a unique and discernible scent, yet it is the combination that makes the heady aroma that is the signature fragrance of the garden. By working and living together in complete co-operation and community, humankind moves forward on a graceful and harmonious path of spiritual evolution and ever-expanding, more beautiful, collaborative creations.

When honored as a living being and treated with respect, compassion, and loving-kindness, Earth grows food abundantly to feed all Her children. Regenerative agriculture, biodynamic farming, organic farming, permaculture, Perelandra gardening,[134] and other ancient and new forms of agriculture that honor Earth are flourishing and feeding all humans high vibrational, nutrient-rich foods. Food gardens, herb gardens, medicinal gardens, wall gardens, vertical gardens, victory gardens, and community gardens are common. Higher life force energy and vitality is contained within all plants. Humans eat a natural, non-GMO, plant-based diet, and there is plenty of pure, nutritious food for all. Higher knowledge about eating animals and ingesting the energies of pain, suffering, and death is common knowledge. With nutritious foods and nourishment from sunlight, illness and disease are rare. Optimal health and well-being are enjoyed by all.

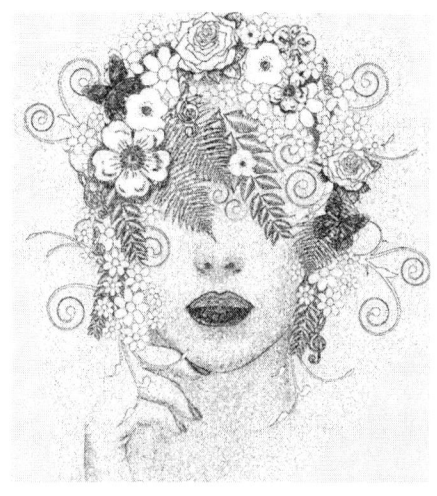

---

[134] Wright, M.S. *Perelandra Garden Workbook: A Complete Guide to Gardening with Nature Intelligences*. Perelandra Ltd. 1 January 1993

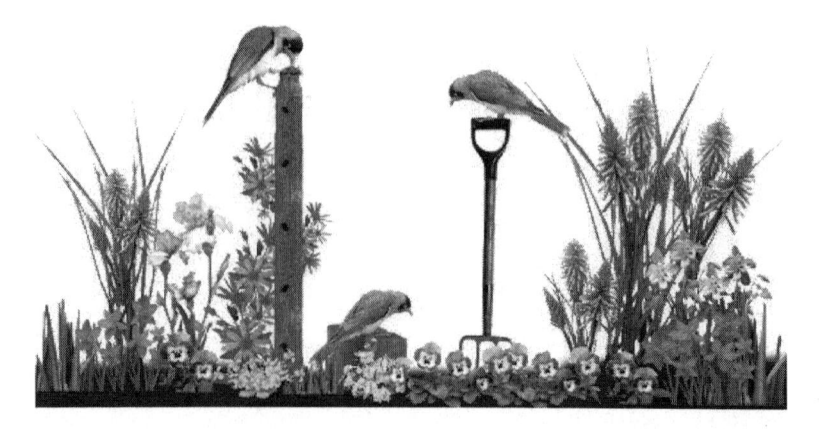

New communities form organically, and existing communities are embellished by new, resonant residents. Clean, free, life-giving energy provides power for all. This energy is beneficial to life. All forms of housing and transport, urban living, work, and recreation combine beauty with functionality. There are cities of light devoted to cultural stimulation, the pursuit of learning, the study and practice of the arts, and the pleasures of community life. There are large and small rural communities. Local governance serves and is subservient to Natural Law and dedicated to the promotion of liberty, prosperity, and the highest good of all. There is not one leader. All may freely and without formality participate to the fullest extent of their capabilities, choices, inclinations, and interests. Guided by the principles of Natural Law, there are no unilateral decisions and no arbitrary justice. There are Upholders of Justice, whose job is not to wield arbitrary authority, but, with the widest public participation, to interpret and apply, as accurately, fairly, and consistently as possible, the guiding rule of right relationships and freedom up to, but never beyond, the point where individual freedom harms or imposes upon the freedom of others.[135]

There is equitable, responsible, and respectful use of natural resources, and a just, stable, and productive basis for economic and commercial activity. Economic, political, and administrative systems support life, promote health and equality, and benefit all. All members serve and are served by their community. Each person contributes to the whole and all basic needs are met. Needs are very simple – food, shelter, clothing, music, movement, meaningful work, loving touch, and kindness – a re-embracing of ancient ways of living. With all basic needs met, there is more time for creativity, spiritual practices, growing food, and enjoying life.

Each community is unique, with its own energetic signature that draws others of like intention. Communities will grow and flourish based on its members' abilities to focus on thought forms together and their willingness to perform actions that serve the greatest good of all. All must want to work together to energize similar thought forms. These thought forms will then create energetic fields that act as magnets for like-intentioned individuals.

Spiritual evolution is central to life. There are many beautiful temples of Light and living Masters and enlightened beings to guide and support individuals through initiations and expansions of consciousness. Initiates learn to befriend the ego, to control the physical body and the non-physical, astral and mental bodies, and to access the Akashic Records

---

[135] Sartorius, L & M. *Book III: Life in the New Age.* www.thenewearth.org 2021 https://thenewearth.org/newearth3.html

and secrets of self-mastery. All contribute to the collective evolution of consciousness.

Babies are lotus-born at home to parents who have healed emotional wounds and studied and prepared for parenthood. Children grow up in a loving, supportive community. Schools educate, not indoctrinate. With the understanding that there are unique ways of processing information, schools accommodate all learning styles. Children learn Natural Law and spiritual truths. They are encouraged and supported to discover and activate their full, Divine potential, to embody, evolve, and employ creative genius, and to make a contribution to the highest good of all. Meditation, critical thinking, galactic history, health promotion, natural medicine, and physical and life skills are taught in school. Children learn how to grow, prepare, and preserve food, make compost, save seeds, and preserve and use medicinal herbs. They learn about fermentation, water filtration and conservation, wild food foraging, and plant medicine. Children learn and practice non-violent communication, conflict resolution, personal responsibility, and autodidacticism.[136] They also learn and practice how to use intuition, telepathy, psychic abilities, clairvoyance, clairaudience, clairsentience, claircognizance,

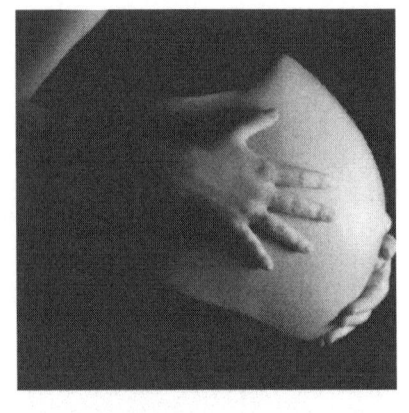

---

[136] Self-education

lucid dreaming, astral travel, intergalactic travel, time travel, bilocation, teleportation, telekinesis, levitation, holographic art and music, crystal geomancy, sacred symbols, music, mathematics, art, and dance. Communication with interdimensional beings and star nations and keys to sacred partnerships and parenting are also taught in schools.

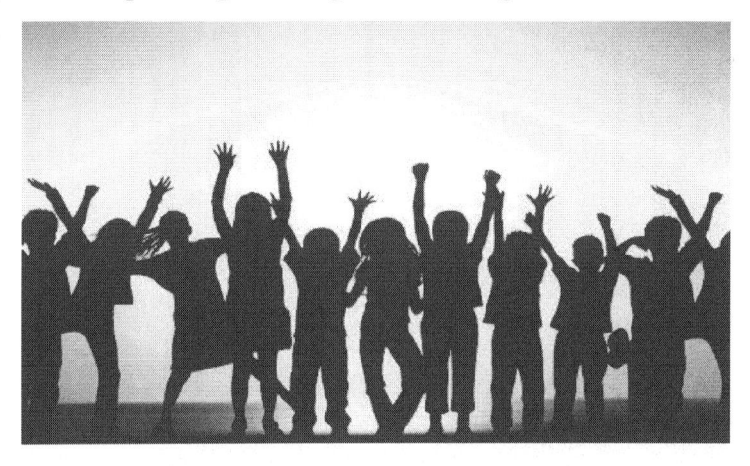

There are new, highly advanced technologies, services, industries, and enterprises that enhance life in the following areas:
- Healthcare
- Land stewardship
- Housing
- Education
- Food production
- Seed banks
- Communication
- Science
- Commerce

- Policing
- Parenting
- Birthing
- Childcare
- Elder Care
- Media
- Dating
- Recreation

Here are some examples...

Travel and Transportation: Free transportation takes travelers wherever they wish to go on a smooth, silent, and time-efficient ride.

Entertainment: Music is uplifting and beneficial to mental and physical health. Movies and books are based on uplifting, life-affirming, and love-based principles.

Healthcare: There are new models for healthcare that are effective and available to all. Healers/doctors practice natural healing and use natural and plant medicines. Both ancient and new healing technologies are freely available. Healing technologies and modalities that have remained hidden are now released. There are healing temples/hospitals that use energy, frequencies, light, color, music, sound, prayer, meditation, movement and food for rejuvenation, regeneration, and to heal any illness and disease, including cures for cancers, regrowth of organs and teeth, and limb replacement. Aging is optional. Lifespan is a personal decision.

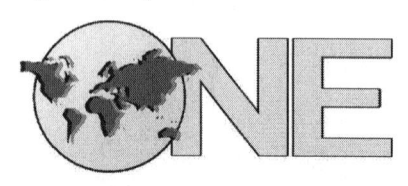

# Signs and Evidence of New Earth

> *"The human drama is reaching its denouement. The great unveiling is approaching, a time when the power structures of the world begin to crumble and people of the heart sing out a new truth. Many voices are joining the chorus, many feet are walking the path, many minds are dreaming possibilities for a magnificent future. For beneath the crises that are looming at every level of civilization, the global heart is awakening, beating out the rhythm of a new and glorious dance, calling us to a better way of living."*
>
> – Anodea Judith

Remember that the more tyrannical governments become and the more egregious, immoral, and outrageous their overreach, the more obvious their deceptions and lies are to more people, and the more power and momentum Truth gains. The more that evil is exposed, witnessed, and experienced by more human beings, the more outraged and activated people become, and the less likely they are to be willing to comply and participate in their own imprisonment. The more people who do not follow orders, the less power those making the rules have and the faster their matrix of control collapses, and the closer we are to living as sovereign beings.

The heartbeat or pulse of Earth, the Schumann Resonance,[137] is registering extremely high frequencies of Light that are literally off the charts. With more Light here, there is more Truth and information available for all. Individual consciousness expands, collective consciousness expands, the frequency of Earth increases and everything with low vibratory energy is no longer sustainable. This time is known as "The Great Quickening" for the following reasons:

- Never-seen levels of electromagnetic frequencies and CMEs (Coronal Mass Ejections) hitting Earth, raising the vibrational frequency of all life on Earth, illuminating evil, and destroying the matrix of mind control.
- Burgeoning numbers of people are realizing they are being lied to and that they cannot trust governments, politicians, doctors, hospitals, police, scientists, celebrities, public education, and mainstream media.

---

[137] All life exists within a sea of vibration. All things vibrate at their own frequency. The Earth vibrates at Her own frequency – the heartbeat of the Earth, the frequency of AUM, the universal sound of Creation, the Schumann Resonance. The Schumann Resonance is the average frequency of the Earth's naturally-generated, electromagnetic frequencies – the electromagnetic waves that circulate between the Earth's surface and the Ionosphere. It is the resonant frequency, the pulse, and the tuning fork for life on Earth. It is typically measured at 7.83 Hz with higher fluctuations over 150 Hz as the vibrational frequency of the planet increases. Earth surrounds and protects all living things with a natural frequency pulsation – Life Force energy. The symphony of evolution is underscored by the frequency of 7.83 Hz. It gives us power, coherence, and courage. It promotes healing and renewal and restores equilibrium and peace. It acts as the background frequency that influences all life on Earth, including the biological circuitry of the mammalian brain and individual and collective consciousness.

- Mushrooming numbers of people turning inward, embracing spirituality, bringing God into the common narrative, and sending a ripple effect of transformational energy throughout the human collective and the Cosmos.
- More people making connections with star people and other benevolent, interdimensional beings.
- Growing numbers of people praying and calling upon ancestors and other benevolent, non-physical beings for help. Help cannot be given unless it is requested.
- Increasing numbers of people participating in worldwide group meditations and sacred ceremonies for freedom and peace.
- Reports of physical experiences of high vibratory energy, including buzzing, ear ringing, tremors, shakes, and ecstasy.
- Reports of personal experiences of sporadic bursts of energy, receipt of downloads of information, and interdimensional encounters.
- Reports of increased intuition, heightened sense of innate knowing, and experiences of shared thoughts.
- Reports of manifestations of all forms of abundance, including health and well-being.
- Reports of dreams being more vivid, futuristic, lucid, precognitive, and didactic.
- Reports of physical experiences of multiple reality overlays, synchronicities, and Divine timing.
- Reports of seeing repeating number patterns, seeing interdimensionally, and remote viewing.

- Reports of out-of-body experiences, sleep paralysis, and astral projection.
- Reports of expedited healing.
- Reports of nails and hair growing faster and hair retuning to original color and growing back.
- Drastic reduction in the slaughter of animals for meat consumption.
- Growing numbers of people disconnecting from the matrix of fear and control and reconnecting with Nature.
- Millions of people are choosing to leave employment and no longer participate in tyranny, wage slavery, and neo-feudalism in record numbers.[138]
- More people simplifying their lives, spending more time outdoors, relocating, downsizing, and moving out of cities in droves.
- More people tuning inward, listening to and following intuition, thinking independently and critically, and nurturing right relationships.
- Quantum physics is replacing Newtonian physics.
- Public demands for truth and transparency are rising.
- More people are undertaking independent research.
- More are people using their platforms to speak, write, create content, and share information to expose official lies, quantifiable fraud, false mainstream narratives and numberfuckery, government hypocrisy, weaponized

---

[138] https://www.nytimes.com/2021/10/12/business/economy/workers-quitting-august.html?smid=tw-nytimes&smtyp=cur

federal agencies, and police brutality.
- Every day more jab victims and their families are flooding social media with their horrifying and heartbreaking stories, images, and videos of injuries and deaths from the shots.
- Information sharing is ballooning despite worldwide, Nazi-type censorship.
- The rise of independent media and citizen journalism.
- Independent news sources are more popular than mainstream news/propaganda.
- Rising mistrust and loss of faith in governments, politicians, police, mainstream media, doctors, hospitals, celebrities, and public education.[139]
- The rise of patriot militias and parallel law enforcement.
- Increasing exposure of maleficence, deception, fraud, and corruption at all levels of government – past and present.
- Rapidly growing, insuppressible, worldwide uprisings and pushback by individuals, groups, unions, businesses, states, and nations against treason, traitors, and totalitarianism.

***Because all totalitarian projects are built upon lies and deception, they hold the seeds of their self-destruction.***

---

[139] https://www.naturalnews.com/2021-09-27-dr-nepute-americans-losing-faith-hospital-system.html

# THE GREAT REBELLION IS WELL UNDERWAY

Burgeoning numbers of people from all countries and all walks of life are showing solidarity, fighting back against the forces of conquest, claiming freedom, taking a stand for freedom, practicing peaceful noncompliance and civil disobedience, and refusing to comply with tyrannical employers, governments, police, military, and a global fascist dictatorship.

Every day more people are taking to the streets to protest government overreach and medical apartheid, which increases personal power, strengthens the bond of dissonant voices, and terrifies our enemy. Rallies, blockades, strikes, and walkouts are increasing worldwide. More people are joining the "A Stand in the Park" movement and are standing together in parks, on roundabouts,[140] and during picnics in parks to celebrate freedom, diversity, and fairness for all.

More people are becoming activists and using their time, energy, resources, money, platforms, keyboards, and creativity to expose deception and corruption – through art, music, videos, campaigns, letter drops, and fact-sharing.

Increasing public outrage, uprisings, walkouts, and growing public demonstrations wherever draconian and unlawful legislation is being voted upon, including political, electoral, and school board meetings.

---

[140] https://astandinthepark.org/
https://rebelsonroundabouts.com/

Whistleblowers and truthtellers from all walks of life (doctors, nurses, teachers, police, scientists, military, politicians, tradesmen) are coming forward to sound the alarm and are speaking out about the lies, deceptions, and evil agendas.

Published research and data analyses on the injection experiment prove these jabs are unsafe, ineffective, and the most deadly of all.

Many who have suffered injuries and their families are speaking out, sharing their stories, using their platforms, and raising the alarm about the fake virus narrative and the dangers of these bioweapons.

> ***Your DNA is the battleground. Protect your humanity and your children at any cost or our future will be lost.***

## THE GREAT RESIGNATION HAS BEGUN

Increasing numbers of people are refusing to compromise their integrity, serve evil, comply with medical tyranny, and support medical apartheid. Multitudes are resigning or being illegally terminated from employment, including doctors, nurses, police, military, judges, teachers, hospitality employees, airline employees, truck drivers, and construction workers. There are no facilities large enough anywhere to contain all freedom warriors who will never comply.

More legal actions are being taken worldwide, including

reporting of crimes against Humanity, and personal and class action lawsuits being filed against government agencies and individuals.

> *"The hunters are starting to get hunted. All the degenerates and devolved pagans who planned and executed the worst crime in history must stand trial before international tribunals. If convicted for crimes against Humanity, they should be executed by lethal injection with the Covid-19 poison death shots. The media, academia, politicians, and industry tyrants who lied and murdered millions should be brought to justice. The Nazi-like physicians who "just followed orders" should be brought to justice. Not vigilante justice but international tribunals. Let the world know and see what happens to sociopathic vermin when they desecrate God's creation. Justice and glorious days of peace are coming."*
>
> – Vladimir Zev Zelenko[141]

More government agencies, hospitals, healthcare organizations, schools, and individuals are being put on notice in more countries. Increasing numbers of judges, politicians, government employees, medical professionals, school boards, school administrators, teachers, police, religious leaders, corporate CEOs, and mainstream media scum are being

---

[141] https://vladimirzelenkomd.com/

served legal documents requesting them to provide proof to validate lockdowns and restriction orders. They are being publicly exposed and shamed and being served with notices of liability for violations of the Nuremberg Code and human rights and being held to account for failing to uphold oaths they have sworn, and for medical rape, unfair dismissal, extortion, treason, genocide, and crimes against Humanity. To avoid consequences for their crimes, political leaders, politicians, government officials, medical professionals, and CEOs are resigning en masse.

Large scale investigations into philanthropic organizations are underway.

Growing numbers of successful legal challenges including national injunctions, to illegal, unconstitutional, and evil government mandates by individuals, unions, sports teams, business owners, and states.

Growing numbers of arrests of corrupt government officials, pedophiles, and human traffickers, which are not being reported by mainstream media.

Increasing numbers of people withdrawing support for major companies, banks, and online platforms – Amazon, Google, Facebook, Twitter, Instagram – and creating new censorship-free, discrimination-free alternatives.

The rise of alternative banking and commerce.

The rise of the bartering economy.

The rise of cryptocurrency and counter economy groups.

Alternative communication systems are being implemented.

***In the event that communications go out, we will all meet at our local libraries, every Saturday at 9am. In every town, city, and in every state. Pass it on.***

More people are losing faith and leaving allopathic medicine *en masse* for alternative, natural, and holistic healthcare options that produce results and help people heal.[142]

The rise of alternative healing clinics and sanctuaries.

More people taking responsibility for creating and maintaining health and reducing dependence upon doctors and pharmaceuticals.

***"According to the WHO, mainstream medicine is 'wobbling.'"***

– AUSTRALIAN VACCINATION-RISKS NETWORK INC.[143]

Doctors and other healthcare professionals leaving mainstream medicine and forming pods of healthcare advocates, establishing healing centers, and offering in-home care.

Alternatives to health insurance.

More parents and child caregivers taking action to protect children, who are the main targets of Big Pharma and government campaigns to get them injected.

---

[142] *Tomey, R. Dr. Eric Nepute: Americans losing faith in the hospital system* – Brighteon.TV. www.naturalnews.com 27 September 2021 https://www.naturalnews.com/2021-09-27-dr-nepute-americans-losing-faith-hospital-system.html

[143] Australian Vaccination-risks Network Inc. (AVN): https://avn.org.au/

Surge in home births. Hundreds of thousands more babies are being born at home, where birthing belongs.

Skyrocketing numbers of children are being withdrawn from public education and are now homeschooled and privately tutored.[144]

More elders are being cared for at home, rather than warehoused, poisoned, and murdered in "care homes."

More people are choosing not to support Amazon, Costco, Walmart, and other pandemic profiteers and choosing to support local businesses and farmers instead. More people are choosing to become more self-sufficient, grow food, live off-grid, in tiny homes, and in intentional communities.

The rise of intentional communities, parallel structures, parallel societies, cohousing, and sufficient communities that celebrate faith, family, and freedom, and the expansion of existing freedom-based, love-based communities.

> ***"One of the most important tasks the 'dissident movements' have set themselves is to support and develop parallel social structures. What else are those initial attempts at social self-organization than the efforts of a certain part of society to rid itself of the self-sustaining aspects of totalitarianism and, thus, to extricate itself radically from its involvement in the***

---

[144] CBN NEWS. *More Americans Deciding to Homeschool Their Children as Many Moms Choose to Stay Home.* www1.cbn.com/cbnnews 8 September 2021 https://www1.cbn.com/cbnnews/us/2021/september/more-americans-deciding-to-homeschool-their-children-as-many-moms-choose-to-stay-home

*totalitarian system. The ultimate phase of this process is the situation in which the official structures simply begin withering away and dying off, to be replaced by new structures that have evolved from 'below' and are put together in a fundamentally different way."*

—Václav Havel

Holistic, nature-based healing centers and communities are taking form.

Non-discriminatory businesses and services are mushrooming.

Resurgence of efforts to heed the wisdom of original, indigenous elders and maintain and preserve indigenous cultures, customs, traditions, and languages.

More people are stepping forward to teach Natural Law, Natural Medicine, and occult wisdom and liberation, and to expose the truth about the enslavement of Humanity in a satanic blood cult.

Growing numbers of countries are removing some/all COVID restrictions, vaccine mandates, "Green" passport requirements, and refusing to implement medical apartheid. (Denmark, Sweden, Norway, Brazil, Croatia, Ireland, Romania, Belgium, Zimbabwe, Venezuela, Nicaragua, Belize, Honduras.)

More countries are banning some/all COVID shots. (Iceland, Ireland, Netherlands, Denmark, Norway, Bulgaria, Japan, Italy, France, and Germany.)

Rising numbers of sanctuary states in the US are litigating, removing, and refusing to implement illegal COVID mandates and Nazi-like passports and/or upholding religious and philosophical exemptions from jabs. (Arizona, Arkansas, Georgia, Florida, Indiana, Idaho, Montana, New Hampshire, North Dakota, Oklahoma, Tennessee, Texas, Utah, New Mexico.)

Growing numbers of hospitals, health clinics, businesses, schools, colleges, universities, churches, airlines, and organizations are rescinding government mandates and refusing to enforce medical apartheid.

Increasing number of cases against COVID impositions, including mask and vaccine mandates, being won in courts worldwide.

Public exposure of the UFO reality and an explosion of sightings and contact with interdimensional peers is rapidly growing.

Everyday more people are maintaining a high vibrational frequency and focusing on visioning, embodying, and co-creating New Earth, which is accelerating the collapse of the old paradigm and ensuring that the rise of New Earth is well underway.

> ***This is the beginning of the end of our enslavement. The speed at which we collapse the old paradigm and build anew is in our hands and hearts. The more that Divine Light/Love is embodied and amplified by individuals, the sooner the mind control matrix is destroyed, and New Earth takes form. For those of us who see the way forward, it is our responsibility to envision, shape, and co-create the future.***

*To co-create a future that is best for a human being, not a cyborg, it is imperative that we stay human, stay grounded, avoid the metaverse, virtual realities, the merging of AI with our bodies, and protect our humanity at all costs. Screen technologies have been designed to capture our attention, disempower us, and distract us from what we are here to do as architects of our future. The more time spent interacting with a screen, the less time one has to become fully empowered. The choice to inhabit the natural world or virtual worlds is the choice between power and powerlessness, freedom and slavery, and our organic timeline and an artificial, transhuman timeline. Which reality and which timeline are you giving your power to?*

What is *your* vision for New Earth?
How are you co-creating New Earth?
What collective magnificent, magical, mathematical, bioelectromagnetic dream are we dreaming for humankind?

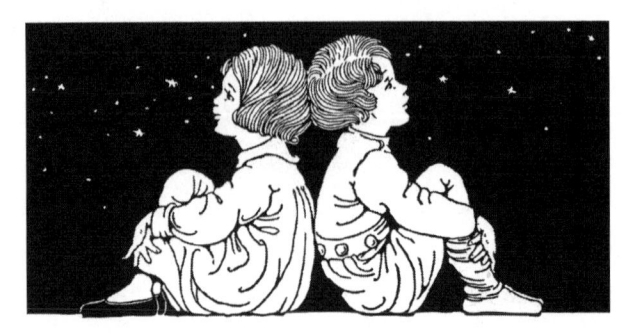

# RESOURCES

# COVID-19 FACTS

Doctors for Covid Ethics: https://doctors4covidethics.org/
PANDA (Pandemics Data Analysis): https://www.pandata.org/team/
FLCCC Alliance (Front Line COVID-19 Critical Care Alliance): https://covid19criticalcare.com/
HART (Health Advisory and Recovery Team): https://www.hartgroup.org/
Children's Health Defense Fund: https://childrenshealthdefense.org/
Covid Medical Network: https://www.covidmedicalnetwork.com/
Millions Against Medical Mandates: www.mamm.org
Americas Frontline Doctors: https://www.americasfrontlinedoctors.org/
World Doctors Alliance: www.worlddoctorsalliance.com
Medscape: https://www.medscape.com/
Health Freedom for Humanity: https://healthfreedomforhumanity.org/
World Freedom Alliance: https://worldfreedomalliance.org/
The Mirror Project: https://www.mp-22.com/
Vaxxed II - The Peoples Truth: https://www.vaxxed2.com/
National Vaccine Information Center: https://www.nvic.org/
VacTruth: www.vactruth.com
Virus-hoax.com: https://virus-hoax.com/

COVID Truths: https://www.covidtruths.co.uk/
Green Med Info: www.greenmedinfo.com
Alliance For Natural Health: www.anhinternational.org/
Yummy-Doctor: https://yummy.doctor/
The Healthy American: https://www.thehealthyamerican.org/
The New Abnormal: https://thenewabnormal513330780.wordpress.com/
Chemical Violence: https://chemicalviolence.com/index.html
No Jab For me: https://nojabforme.info/#startenglish
Vaxxter: https://vaxxter.com/
COVID-19 UNCENSORED: https://thevirus.wtf/
Vaccine Impact: https://vaccineimpact.com/
VaxTruth: vaxtruth.org

# DOCTORS UPHOLDING THE HIPPOCRATIC OATH

Dr. Robert Malone (Inventor of mRNA and DNA vaccine technology): https://www.rwmalonemd.com/about-us
Dr. Geert Vanden Bossche: https://www.geertvandenbossche.org/
Dr. Peter McCullough: www.americaoutloud.com
Dr. Tess Lawrie: https://www.e-bmc.co.uk/
Dr. Simone Gold: https://thegoldopinion.com/
Dr. Christiane Northrup: https://www.drnorthrup.com/
Dr. Sherri Tenpenny: https://www.drtenpenny.com/
Dr. Lee Merritt - The Medical Rebel: https://drleemerritt.com/

Dr. Stephanie Seneff: https://stephanieseneff.net/
Dr. Larry Palevsky: https://www.northportwellnesscenter.com/
Dr. Shiva Ayyadurai: https://vashiva.com/
Dr. Amandha Vollmer: https://yummy.doctor/
Dr. Joseph Mercola: https://www.mercola.com/
Dr. Carrie Madej: https://carriemadej.com/
Dr. Michael Yeadon: #DrMichaelYeadon
Dr. Judy Mikovits: https://drjudyamikovits.com/
Dr. Jane Ruby: http://drjaneruby.com/
Dr. Geert Vanden Bossche: https://www.geertvandenbossche.org/
Dr. Mark Sircus: https://drsircus.com/
Dr. Andrew Kaufman: https://andrewkaufmanmd.com/
Dr. Dolores Cahill: https://dolorescahill.com/
Dr. Christine Stabell Benn: Bandim Health Project https://www.bandim.org/
Dr. Roger Hodkinson: https://medmaldoctors.ca/medmaldoctors/
Dr. Heiko Schoning: https://worlddoctorsalliance.com/
Dr. Suzanne Humphries: http://bit.ly/17sKDbf
Dr. Russell Blaylock: http://bit.ly/1BXxQZL
Dr. Rashid Buttar: https://www.drbuttar.com/
Dr. Pierre Kory: FLCCC Alliance. https://covid19criticalcare.com/
Dr. Scott Jensen: https://drscottjensen.com/
Dr. Vernon Coleman: www.vernoncoleman.org
Professor Sucharit Bhakdi: https://sucharitbhakdi.de/
Dr. Astrid Stuckleberger: https://www.astridstuckelberger.com/

Dr. Gary G. Khols: http://www.mindbodymedicineduluth.com/index.html
Dr. Ben Tapper: https://www.thewellnesspointe.com/
Dr. Eric Nepute: https://neputewellnesscenter.com/about/
Dr. Nancy Banks: http://bit.ly/1lp0alm
Dr. Shiv Chopra: http://bit.ly/1gdgh1s
Dr. Vladimir (Zev) Zelenko: https://vladimirzelenkomd.com/
Dr Bryan Ardis: https://thedrardisshow.com/

# PROTOCOLS FOR HEALING, DETOXIFICATION, AND PROTECTION

Dr. Zelenko COVID-19 Treatment Protocol: https://vladimirzelenkomd.com/treatment-protocol/

Dr Bryan Ardis Disease Prevention Protocol: https://files.elfsightcdn.com/5266f37f-1e60-4e3b-9202-0f9e41473266/671419ba-2179-4db4-a924-cde7c8fdb97c.pdf

David (Avocado) Wolfe Protection Protocol: https://rightsfreedoms.wordpress.com/2021/09/13/summary-of-the-spike-protein-protocol-protection-against-spike-protein-and-vaccine-shedding-contagion-from-vaccinated-persons/

Clif High Vax Repair Protocol:
Wilson, A. BREAKING NEWS: Clif High With "Vaccine Repair Protocol." www.thetruedefender.com. 2 September 2021 https://thetruedefender.com/breaking-news-clif-high-with-vaccine-repair-protocol/

World Council For Health. *Spike Protein Detox Guide.* www.worldcouncilforhealth.org 2 December 2021

https://worldcouncilforhealth.org/resources/spike-protein-detox-guide/
Gene Decode's Vax Detox Protocol: https://awakeneduk.wordpress.com/2021/09/19/gene-decodes-vax-detox-protocol/
Richardson, K. *Graphene Oxide – How to eradicate it.* www.new-earth-healing.com. 7 September 2021 https://www.new-earth-healing.com/blog/graphene-oxide-how-to-eradicate-it
Love, A. *Graphene Oxide Detox Protocols For The Vaxxed and Unvaxxed.* www.ambassadorlove.wordpress.com 21 October 2021 https://ambassadorlove.wordpress.com/2021/08/24/graphene-oxide-detox-protocols-for-the-vaxxed-and-unvaxxed/
KatrinaH. *Nutrition Protocols To Deactivate & Neutralize Graphene Oxide.* www.katrinah.com https://katrinah.com/nutrition-protocol-to-neutralize-graphene-oxide/

## DATABASES THAT RECORD DEATHS AND ADVERSE REACTIONS TO ALL JABS:

PLEASE REPORT ANY ADVERSE REACTIONS.
VAERS (Vaccine Adverse Event Reporting System); www.VAERS.org
Open VAERS: https://www.openvaers.com/index.php VAERS Covid Vax Records: https://vaxpain.us/
The COVID Tracking Project: https://covidtracking.com/about

Doctors Report Adverse Events: https://www.medscape.com/sites/public/covid-19/vaccine-insights/how-concerned-are-you-about-vaccine-related-adverse-events

C19 Vax reactions: https://www.c19vaxreactions.com/

Covid Vaccine Victims: https://www.covidvaccinevictims.com/

Yellow Card Scheme: https://yellowcard.mhra.gov.uk/

https://www.gov.uk/government/publications/coronavirus-covid-19-vaccine-adverse-reactions/coronavirus-vaccine-summary-of-yellow-card-reporting

UK Company Reaction to COVID-19: www.covidreactions.com

EudraVigilance – European Database of suspected adverse drug reaction reports:

https://www.adrreports.eu/en/index.html

Australian Therapeutic Goods Administration:

https://www.tga.gov.au/reporting-problems

https://www.tga.gov.au/database-adverse-event-notifications-daen

Covid 19 Studies: https://c19early.com/

Report menses irregularities:

www.mycyclestory.com:

www.risemamarise.com

## NEWS SOURCES

HELP WARN THE WORLD!

Educate-Yourself: The Freedom of Knowledge. The Power of Thought

https://educate-yourself.org/

Want To Know: https://www.wanttoknow.info/

Project Veritas: https://www.projectveritas.com/news/
Hardline Investigative Report: www.americanmediaperiscope.com
Catherine Austin Fitts: Solari Report
https://home.solari.com/
James Corbet: www.thecorbettreport.com
The HighWire:
https://thehighwire.com/watch/
From the Trenches World Report:
https://fromthetrenchesworldreport.com/
News Rescue: https://newsrescue.com/
Not The Beeb: https://www.notonthebeeb.co.uk/home2
Clif_High:
https://www.bitchute.com/channel/HBBwqd0My7Gz/
The Daily Expose: https://dailyexpose.co.uk/
Dark Journalist: The Truth Runs Deep.
https://www.darkjournalist.com/
We Are The Change: https://wearechange.org/
Red Voice Media: https://www.redvoicemedia.com/
Timcast: https://timcast.com/news/
A Warrior Calls: https://awarriorcalls.com/
Elana Freeland: https://www.elanafreeland.com/
Bret Weinstein - Darkhorse podcast: https://bretweinstein.net/
In Defense of Humanity: https://indefenseofhumanity.com/
Mission Possible World Health International:
http://www. mpwhi.com/main.htm
Truth Unmasked: www.truthunmasked.org
Forbidden Knowledge: www.forbiddenknowledgetv.net
Natural News: www.naturalnews.com
Make Americans Free Again: https://makeamericansfreeagain.

com/
The Last American Vagabond: https://www.thelastamericanvagabond.com/
Clay Clark: www.timetofreeamerica.com
Stand For Freedom: www.standforhealthfreedom.com
Freedom Coalition: https://www.freedomco.net/videos
The Daily Wire: https://www.dailywire.com/

# ACTIVISM

Great Barrington Declaration: https://gbdeclaration.org/
Stop World Control: https://www.stopworldcontrol.com/
Project Veritas: https://www.projectveritas.com/
Veritas Radio: https://veritasradio.com/
Millions Against Medical Mandates: www.mamm.org
Americas Frontline Doctors: https://www.americasfrontlinedoctors.org/
World Doctors Alliance: www.worlddoctorsalliance.com
Medscape: https://www.medscape.com/
Health Freedom for Humanity: https://healthfreedomforhumanity.org/
World Freedom Alliance: https://worldfreedomalliance.org/
Stand For Health Freedom: https://standforhealthfreedom.com/
The Mirror Project: https://www.mp-22.com/
Prepare For Change: https://prepareforchange.net/
The Thrive Movement: http://www.thrivemovement.com/
Enough Movement: https://enoughmovement.org/
Together: https://togetherdeclaration.org/

US Freedom Flyers: https://www.usfreedomflyers.org/
Forbidden Knowledge TV: https://forbiddenknowledgetv.net/
For Our Rights: https://hawaii.forourrights.org/
National Liberty Alliance: https://www.nationallibertyalliance.org/
Vaxxed II - The Peoples Truth: https://www.vaxxed2.com/
National Vaccine Information Center: https://www.nvic.org/
VacTruth: www.vactruth.com
Virus-hoax.com: https://virus-hoax.com/
COVID Truths: https://www.covidtruths.co.uk/
Green Med Info: www.greenmedinfo.com
Alliance For Natural Health: www.anhinternational.org/
Yummy-Doctor: https://yummy.doctor/
The Defender: Children's Health Defense: https://childrenshealthdefense.org/defender/
The New Abnormal: https://thenewabnormal513330780.wordpress.com/
Chemical Violence: https://chemicalviolence.com/index.html
No More Silence: https://nomoresilence.world/
No Jab For me: https://nojabforme.info/#startenglish
Vaxxter: https://vaxxter.com/
COVID-19 UNCENSORED: https://thevirus.wtf/
Voices of Freedom: https://www.voicesforfreedom.co.nz/
Global COVID Summit: https://globalcovidsummit.org/
Vaccine Impact: https://vaccineimpact.com/
The Australia Project: https://theaustraliaproject.org/
Make Australia Healthy Again: https://makeaustraliahealthyagain.org/

Advocate Me: https://www.advocateme.com.au/Australians Against Mandatory Vaccination:
https://www.australianssayno.com/
Canadian COVID Care Alliance:
https://www.canadiancovidcarealliance.org/
COVID Medical Network: https://covidmedicalnetwork.com/
Silent Majority: https://www.silentmajority.co.uk/
In This Together: https://inthistogetheramerica.org/
Geoengineering Watch: https://www.geoengineeringwatch.org/
Our World In Data: https://ourworldindata.org/

## EXEMPTION FORMS

Department of Homeland Security: https://www.dhs.gov
www.dhs.gov/sites/default/files/publications/dhs-medical-exemption-form_11-03-2021.pdf
The Healthy American: https://www.thehealthyamerican.org/
Rumble: *Andy Wakefield | How to Avoid Taking the COVID-19 Vaccines!!!?* Thrivetime Show: Business School without the BS. 4 August 2021
https://rumble.com/vkpqr3-andy-wakefield-how-to-avoid-taking-the-covid-19-vaccines.html
Download the employee COVID-19 exemption form at www.Team1986.com.

## RELIGIOUS EXEMPTIONS

Department of Homeland Security: https://www.dhs.gov

www.dhs.gov/sites/default/files/publications/dhs-religious-exemption-form_11-03-2021.pdf
The Healthy American:
https://www.thehealthyamerican.org/religious-exemptions
Gab - Download COVID Vaccine Religious Exemption Documents
https://news.gab.com/2021/07/29/important-download-covid-vaccine-religious-exemption-documents-here/

## ATTORNEYS FIGHTING UNLAWFUL MANDATES

There are law firms that you may contact if you believe your rights are being infringed upon by your employer, school, college, or any group that discriminates against you for not complying with their vaccine or mask mandates. Mount legal challenges and fight all transgressions of your rights with all means available. Make it costly in time and money for employers and business owners to violate human rights.

These websites offer excellent legal resources:
Daily News of America
https://dailyusa24.com/2021/09/06/breaking-us-courts-website-publishes-list-of-vaccine-attorneys-to-fight-dangerous-vaccines/
Constitutional Law Group:
https://www.constitutionallawgroup.us/
Liberty Counsel: https://lc.org/
Liberty Institute: https://www.libertyinstitute.org/about/faq
Pacific Justice Institute: https://pacificjustice.org/

Advocates For Faith and Freedom: https://faith-freedom.com/
Alliance Defending Freedom: https://adflegal.org/about-us
National Legal Foundation: https://nationallegalfoundation.org/
Thomas More Law Center: https://www.thomasmore.org/
Thomas More Society: https://thomasmoresociety.org/
Christian Legal Society: https://www.christianlegalsociety.org/
American Center for Law and Justice: https://aclj.org/
Center for Law and Religious Freedom: https://www.clsreligiousfreedom.org/about-center
Christian Attorneys of America: https://christianattorneysofamerica.com/
Christian Law Association: https://www.christianlaw.org/
National Association of Christian Lawmakers: https://christianlawmakers.com/
Pacific Legal Foundation: https://pacificlegal.org/
Advocate Me: https://www.advocateme.com.au/
Lawyers For Liberty: https://lawyersforliberty.uk/
Class Action:
Peter & Maatouks Law Group: https://callpeter.com.au/

# ESCAPE THE MATRIX OF CONTROL

Methods of Claiming your Straw Man: https://www.newhumannewearthcommunities.com/methods-of-claiming-your-strawman
Claim Your Strawman: https://www.claimyourstrawman.com/optin1631368380241

Escaping the Matrix: 8 Ways to Deprogram Yourself:
https://sofoarchon.com/deprogramming/
YouTube: *How to Escape from a Sick Society*. Academy of Ideas.
7 September 2021.
https://www.youtube.com/watch?v=JeliRVZ4V00

## NATURAL LAW

https://www.whatonearthishappening.com/
https://onegreatworknetwork.com/

## COMMON LAW

Common Law Courts: https://www.commonlawcourt.com/
Common Law: https://commonlaw.earth/
A Warrior Calls: https://awarriorcalls.com/
Australian Peoples's Governance: https://ausreal.net/
The Australia Project: https://theaustraliaproject.org

## NEW EARTH COMMUNITIES

New Humane New Earth Communities:
https://www.newhumannewearthcommunities.com/
New Earth Community: https://newearth.community/
The New Earth: https://thenewearth.org/
New Earth Network: https://newearth.network/
New Earth Living: https://www.newearthliving.com.au/

# ALTERNATIVE LIFESTYLES

Off grid living: https://offgridliving.net/
Off Grid World: https://offgridworld.com/
Tiny homes: https://parkmytinyhouse.com.au/
Foundation for Intentional Communities: https://www.ic.org/
Free State Project: https://www.fsp.org/
Boondocking: https://boondocking.org/

# SUSTAINABLE FOOD PRODUCTION AND LAND STEWARDSHIP

Regenerative agriculture: https://sustainableamerica.org/blog/what-is-regenerative-agriculture/
Permaculture: https://epdf.pub/permaculture-a-designers-manual.html
Biodynamic gardening: https://www.biodynamics.com/
Perelandra gardening: Wright, M.S. *Perelandra Garden Workbook: A Complete Guide to Gardening with Nature Intelligences.* Perelandra Ltd. 1 January 1993
Findhorn Foundation: https://www.findhorn.org/about-us/
Reko Rings[145]
Retrosuburbia[146]

---

[145] https://www.corbettreport.com/solutionswatch-reko/

[146] https://www.researchgate.net/

Ripe Near Me: https://www.ripenear.me/
Local Harvest: https://www.localharvest.org/
Foodscaping and agrihoods in urban environments.

## NONVIOLENT COMMUNICATION

Rosenberg. M. *Nonviolent Comminucation: A Language of Life*. Puddledancer Press. USA. 2003.
https://www.nonviolentcommunication.com/

## NATURAL BIRTHING

Homebirth. Free Birth. Natural Birth. Love-based Birth. Birthing centers.
Birth Freedom: https://www.birthfreedom.com.au/
Lotus Birth: http://www.lotusbirth.net/
Midwifery: https://www.midwife.org/
Doulas: https://www.dona.org/

## EDUCATION MODELS

Waldorf Education: https://www.waldorfeducation.org/waldorf-education
Steiner Education Australia: https://www.steinereducation.edu.au/
Montessori Schools:

---

publication/323986370_Retrosuburbia_the_downshifters_guide_to_a_resilient_future

https://montessori-nw.org/about-montessori-education
Homeschooling and homeschooling co-ops:
https://teachbesideme.com/
how-to-start-a-homeschool-co-op/
Kroka: https://kroka.org/
Green School: https://www.greenschool.org/
Free School (Unschooling): Cowden, F. et al. *Life is the School, Love is the Lesson: An adventure in free schooling.* CreateSpace Independent Publishing Platform. 6 April 2012.
Private Education Association:
https://sourcepma.com/private-education-association/

## DISCRIMINATION-FREE BUSINESSES

Open For All: https://www.openforall.com.au/
All Welcome Here: https://www.allwelcomehere.com.au/
Reignite Democracy Australia:
https://www.reignitedemocracyaustralia.com.au/

## DISCRIMINATION-FREE JOB MARKET WEBSITES AND SOCIAL MEDIA PLATFORMS:

No Vax Mandate Job Board: https://novaxmandate.org/
Jab Free Jobs: https://www.jabfreejobs.info/
NoVaxJobsUSA.com: https://novaxjobsusa.com/
Freedom Job Network:
https://www.thefreedomjobnetwork.com/
No Jab Jobs: https://timetofreeamerica.com/no-jab-jobs/

RedBalloon: https://redballoon.work/
Wise Minds: https://wiseminds.com.au
All Welcome Here: https://www.allwelcomehere.com.au
Free Jobs: https://www.freejobs.com.au/
Open For All: https://www.openforall.com.au/
https://oneandfreeaussie.com/classifieds/browse-ads/82/homeschooling/
https://oneandfreeaussie.com/business-directory/
https://www.reignitedemocracyaustralia.com.au/business-directory/

## TELEGRAM:

https://t.me/freejobsaustralia
https://t.me/jobswithoutjabsaustralia
https://t.me/AustraliaJobsNoVaxNeeded
https://t.me/unvaxxedfriendlybizdirectory
https://t.me/NSWBusinessUnitedDirectory
https://t.me/australia_business_group
https://t.me/businesseswhowelcomeall

## FACEBOOK GROUPS:

Jobs without Jabs:
https://www.facebook.com/groups/1509592039393693/?ref=share
https://www.facebook.com/groups/1213829215752696/?ref=share

Do your own research. Search online for discrimination-free websites, platforms, and apps (such as GAB) for:
Accommodation
Dating
Dining out
Entertainment
Wellness professionals
Tradesmen and women

For example, here are two resources for Travel and Bartering:
Travel:
Freedom Travel Alliance:
https://www.freedomtravelalliance.com/
Traveling Lifestyle:
https://www.travelinglifestyle.net/countries-without-covid-travel-restrictions-no-test-no-quarantine/

Bartering: LETS (Local Exchange Trading System; Local Energy Transfer System).
Community Exchange System.

***Thank you for your contribution to the freedom and future of Humanity.***

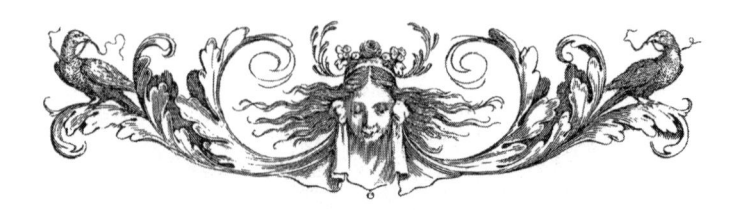

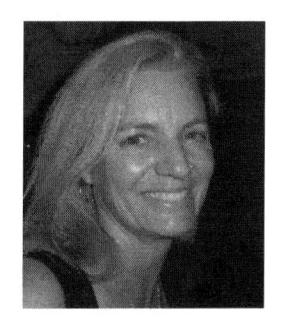

Isabella Young (B.Ed., M.Ed. Pre.) studied and taught Physical Education, Outdoor Education, Health, and Exercise Physiology to undergraduate and postgraduate students in Victoria, Australia. She was a pioneer in the establishment, development, and research of therapeutic Outdoor Education programs in Australia, and a founder of Out Doors Inc. (www.outdoorsinc.org.au), a non-profit organization that has provided outdoor adventure and recreation programs for people with poor mental health since 1987.

In 1994, while completing a Ph.D. and lecturing in Outdoor Education, personal tragedy struck. At 33, widowed, pregnant, and with a three-year-old son, Isabella began her own healing journey that has spanned three decades. She has crisscrossed three continents under three different names, undertaking pilgrimages, retreats, shamanic journeys, and vision quests; living in the wilderness and in ashrams, including eight years in a messianic cult as the wife of the "guru," who took the life of her son to prevent being exposed as a pedophile, a rapist, a thief, and a con man. Her son's murder broke her free from brainwashing, and she escaped to Hawaii. Through her relentless devotion to heal, free her mind, and discover Truth, Isabella is now free from cult programming and suffering and enjoying life immersed in the natural beauty of Kauai, writing, swimming, growing food, and going barefoot.

In 2022 Isabella will release the second book in this series, *Protection From Bioweaponry* and *Feeling Better Naturally:*

*Medicines for the Great Awakening and the Future of Humanity*, which is essential reading to understand that all that we need for optimal health and well-being is found within our physical body, within Nature, and within our Divine nature. This book is replete with information that supports sovereignty and self-empowerment, including hundreds of natural medicines that promote optimal spiritual, mental, physical, and world health. Isabella's articles on natural health appear in *For Kaua'i* and *The Mother* magazines. The short story of her daughter's natural birth is published in *Lotus Birth: Leaving the Umbilical Cord Intact*. Her digital artwork, *Divine In Nature*, accompanies the meditations in *The Secret Garden: Creative Visualizations in the Sanctuary of the Heart*.

For more information, please visit:<br>
www.feelingbetternaturally.love<br>
Facebook: Isabella Young<br>
YouTube: Feeling Better Naturally<br>
https://www.youtube.com/channel/<br>
UCuqQ9wyDhecHBf0WAZ42E4A<br>
Bitchute: Feeling Better Naturally<br>
https://www.bitchute.com/channel/7MuOhOhnDGNl/<br>
Telegram: https://t.me/joinchat/WLfUTyX_iVY5OWVh<br>
Odysee: https://odysee.com/@FeelingBetterNaturally:5<br>
Contact: isabellayoung19@gmail.com

If this book was beneficial in any way, please leave a review on Amazon. I read every review, and they help new readers discover the book and empower themselves. Thank you.

Printed in Great Britain
by Amazon